May 10, 1987

Lindy Neuhaus

It's Okay, God, We Can Take It

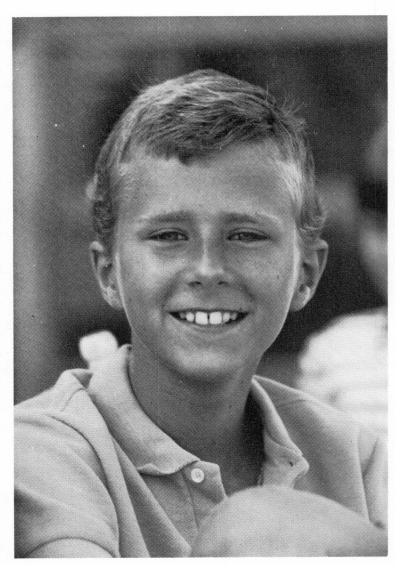

Bo Neuhaus, June 1984

It's Okay, God, We Can Take It

Bo Neuhaus

With
Laura (Lindy) Wyatt-Brown Neuhaus

EAKIN PRESS ☆ Austin, Texas

Library of Congress Cataloging-in-Publication Data

Neuhaus, Bo, 1973–1985.
    It's okay, God, we can take it.

    1. Neuhaus, Bo, 1973–1985 — Health. 2. Liver — Cancer —
Patients — Texas — Biography. 3. Sarcoma — Patients — Texas —
Biography.   I Title.
RC280.L5N486   1986   248.8'6'0924 [B]   86-16513
ISBN 0-89015-576-3

*Dedicated to the glory of
God for the love He has shown us
through our family and friends.
And also to Mary Kessler, Charlie, and Ali.*

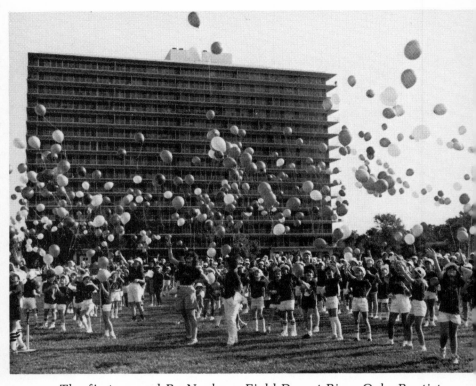

The first annual Bo Neuhaus Field Day at River Oaks Baptist School, May 1985.

It's Okay, God, We Can Take It *is a book written by a very special twelve-year-old boy, Laurence Bosworth Neuhaus, Jr., who had liver cancer for two and one-half years. From the time he was diagnosed in December of 1982, he said he would beat this thing — either in this life or the next. Either way was okay with him. He was never afraid.*

Bo, as he was affectionately called, wanted to write of his experiences for several reasons. First of all, he hoped to help any other children (or adults) who might be in his same position. He combines his understanding of the medical aspects, his terrific sense of humor, and his deep spiritual convictions and faith. He also hoped to bring his readers closer to God. He felt the power of the Holy Spirit carry him through his three surgeries, two years of chemotherapy with all of its side effects, and finally his physical decline. And he wanted people to know the power and love of God as he knew it. He wanted to show people that even though one may face hard times in life, he can still laugh and enjoy life if he maintains a positive attitude.

Bo truly believed that God's plan is a perfect plan, and there was no reason to question it. With God's help, Bo took a wretched situation and turned it into a beautiful and special two years with a glorious ending. He taught many people, his family included, how to live life and realize what is really important on this earth.

This is Bo's story, in a progressive account beginning with his diagnosis. His courageous and uplifting words are supplemented with comments by another who learned about living in the face of death, his mother, Lindy Neuhaus.

v

Contents

Foreword

Bo Neuhaus's story, *It's Okay, God, We Can Take It,* is a book about a warm, loving family and how they faced a killing cancer. The thing that makes this story very unusual is that Bo, a twelve-year-old, had a great faith and led his family and extended family through this very difficult period.

This book is written by Bo and his mother, Lindy Neuhaus. It is more than a textbook about how to face death — although we can learn a lot from it. It is an inspiration and a testimony of great faith. We only met Bo one very brief time, but we will always remember him. You see, Bo did *not* die — Bo went to be with Our Father.

BARBARA AND GEORGE BUSH

Preface

Bo Neuhaus was diagnosed as having a mesenchymal sarcoma of the liver in December 1982 when he was ten years old. This form of cancer is highly malignant, and little effective therapy is currently available. Despite multiple surgical and chemotherapeutic attempts to control his disease, Bo died thirty-nine months later.

However, this narrative is not about the technical aspects of Bo's battle with cancer. Rather, through the eyes of a ten-year-old boy, this narrative envisions what we should all recognize as the truly meaningful qualities in life. This is a story about love and laughter, fear and hope, and, unfortunately, about expectations and compromises. In an age when the sanctity of marriage and the home is under assault, this is a story about family.

And, this is a story about an unshakable faith in God, and trust in His wisdom, mercy, and love. Throughout Bo's narrative, one can see the unfolding of the ideal Christian. Bo's life was an embodiment of St. Paul's words, "We exult in affliction knowing that affliction brings endurance, and endurance tried virtue, and tried virtue hope. And hope does not disappoint because the charity of God is poured forth in our hearts." (Romans 5:3–5)

For families of children with serious chronic or life-threatening illnesses, and even for those who are sometimes overwhelmed by life's inequities, I strongly recommend this book. No one who reads this story can remain untouched nor, having been touched, can fail to reach out and touch someone else in need. Bo's indomitable faith and hope can nurture us all and show us the way to a better life.

DONALD H. MAHONEY, M.D.
Assistant Professor of Pediatrics
Baylor College of Medicine

Introduction

(Written in March 1985, two weeks before Bo died)

For two years I have thought about writing this but somehow I could never make myself sit down and do it. Now as I watch my son, Bo, going steadily downhill still in his battle with cancer, I feel that I have so much to say, so much to be grateful for, and though I get exhausted and frustrated and sometimes angry, I still have a joy and peace in my heart that tells me that it is going to be okay.

I am thirty-seven years old. I have been married for fifteen years to a really special person who is pretty much my best friend. Our relationship is and has always been one based around humor — we love to laugh with each other. We have four children, with whom we also love to laugh. For thirteen of our fifteen years our lives were perfect. Of course, we didn't know that they were perfect back then; we had our normal complaints about dishwashers that didn't work and his being late from work and my forgetting to pick up his shirts at the laundry. Really "important" things, that's what we had to complain about.

We did have one major event in our lives that got our attention. Alexandra, our fourth and final child, was very ill at birth and there were a couple of weeks that we thought she wasn't going to make it. We called her our little "miracle baby" because she had been a critically ill newborn. We became extremely aware of prayer and of God during those weeks and were extremely grateful that she not only survived but could be a normal, bouncing baby.

1

I must add that each of my older sisters had lost a child before this. One was a full-term infant who had so many anomalies that there was no way that any of them could have been corrected; the other, a one-year-old, was a victim of crib death. So when Alexandra was born and was so sick, I simply figured it was my turn.

I am the daughter of a retired Episcopal priest, so obviously I was raised with my share of religion. But I must admit I did not learn to really walk with God or to realize His love and power in my everyday life. I had many blessings as a child but probably didn't recognize them as gifts from God, only matters of circumstance or plain luck.

The two years in which we have been battling my son's cancer have been an emotional roller coaster. Our news has varied from extremely bad to not-so-bad. But I have to say, it has not been without many wonderful blessings and many revelations of God Himself. The fact that I took Bo to the doctor the very first day at 4:30 in the afternoon, fighting Houston traffic (no easy task in itself) instead of my usual waiting until more symptoms appeared, was God's first indication that He was going to lead us through this thing. Had I waited another week or two, a different outcome might have occurred. (With his particular type of cancer, weeks could have mattered.)

The first week, with all the tests and the surgery, was pretty much a fog. The thing I remember most was the outpouring of love and caring from friends, some of whom I didn't know I had. We received hundreds of letters from people wanting to share in our burden. That was very reassuring. We were given many books, some medical, some religious, and some philosophical. Some we read and some we shelved until we could get to them.

After Bo's first surgery, we were told that the tumor they removed from his liver was labeled an undifferentiated mesenchymal hepatic sarcoma. It was a rare and deadly type; so rare that the doctors were only able to come up with sixty cases and only two survivors. And those two survivors were still classified as high risk as the recurrence is almost inevitable. Because it was such a rare type, there was also very little literature on it and drug therapy was strictly experimental — a guessing game, so we were warned. The day we took Bo home from the hospital our surgeon sympathetically told us that he thought we would probably have one good month and then Bo would probably go downhill from there.

Going home with the thought that our time was extremely limited, we had to do some fast thinking because Bo was going to start asking questions and he is not one to miss a trick. How does one tell his child that he may have only two months to live? A pretty horrifying question.

Fortunately (and again I can't believe it was coincidence) Bo was enrolled in a Christian school, River Oaks Baptist Church School, where he had been studying the Bible since first grade. He knew (and still does) a lot more than I, even though I had joined many housewives in taking Bible study classes. We discovered that he had a remarkable Christian foundation.

So we began our discussions about death and what we could expect in the next life. Elizabeth Sinclair, whose child had died of a brain tumor the week that Bo was diagnosed, told me of the conversations she had had with Suzannah about death, and I related many of these truths to Bo. But by the way these words came to me and the ease I found in talking about death, I have to believe that God was right there spurring me on. I told Bo that there was no reason for Christians to be afraid of death. From the moment we are born we begin dying. The only thing that we might be afraid of is the pain of getting to death, but even that could be controlled. We talked about how one thinks about darkness when thinking about death, but Jesus can take that fear away as He is called "the light of the world." We talked about how the time any of us had left on this earth should be utilized getting to know God. Death would be like going to spend the night with one's best friend, and the better one knows his best friend, the more comfortable he will be when he arrives at that friend's house. As I talked to Bo about this, I have to admit I was convincing myself as well as him. I had to *believe* and to *know* that someone more capable than I would be taking care of my little boy in the not-so-far future. Had I not had this belief, I don't think I could have stood the thought of losing my precious child.

I truly learned the meaning of grace. A feeling of peace seemed to come over me and stay with me.

— Lindy

December 1982

It was another dull day. I got home from school and threw my books on the floor and sat on the stairs. My mom came down and said, "How was your day at school?"

I said, "Okay, but I have a stomach ache and my head feels hot."

"Let me take your temperature," she said.

When she went to get the thermometer, I went up to my room. After she took my temperature, she said, "100 degrees, let's go to the doctor."

"Why?" I asked.

She just said, "Come on."

The doctor did a lot of tests on me. He told me not to go to school the next day. I was happy!

The next day was not fun at all. All we did was go back to the doctor and have some more tests done. After that we went back home.

A few hours later my telephone rang. It was the doctor telling mother to take me to Texas Children's Hospital.

I was very scared. "What's happening to me?" I thought to myself. I began to cry.

"It's going to be okay," my mom said.

I said, "No, it's not. I know something bad is going to happen."

When we finally arrived at the hospital, we had to wait in the hall until they called us into a small room.

The man asked, "What is your name?"

I said, "Bo Neuhaus."

He told me to lie down on a table that looked like an operating table. Then he put jelly stuff on my stomach. Then he put a stick on my stomach and moved it around. The man told us to come back the next day.

So we came back the next day. This time they put me in a hospital room. We waited until about 3:00 and then they called us in to a big room. They took x-ray pictures of me. At 5:00, we went home.

The doctor told us to rest up, because on Monday morning I had to come back and have something called an arteriogram. That is when the doctor puts a needle in your leg and can see if you have a tumor.

The thought of a needle scared me, but when they said they were going to put me to sleep, I freaked out with a capital F!

The next morning was Saturday. I was glad because I was very tired.

I had a lot of visitors and gifts. One of the visitors was Gifford Nielsen, the Houston Oilers' quarterback. When my uncle John first told me that Giff was at my house I did not believe him, but when I went downstairs I could not believe it. He was actually at my house! I stood against the wall not knowing what to say.

He put out his hand and said, "Hi, I'm Archie Manning," which is the Oilers' other quarterback. (At that time there was a big rivalry between Giff and Archie Manning to be the number one quarterback.)

I said, "Huh?" not expecting him to say that.

Everybody laughed except for me. I did not know what was going on. Then I laughed too. He told us all about being with the Oilers. That was a fun day.

On Sunday night we had to go back to the hospital. I was very scared. When we got there, I had a visitor. It was my dad's uncle, Laurence. He was very nice. We had fun.

The next day was not fun. The only thing we did that I loved was praying for God's help. We were not very good at praying, but that does not matter because God understands everything you say and He loves you.

The next thing that happened was terrible. They gave me a shot in my seat.

I screamed, "Help!"

All of a sudden I started to feel sleepy. The next thing I knew, I was on the operating table.

I still was very tired. I was trying to pray my hardest. It was no use. Then I felt myself drift off to sleep.

When I woke up, I did not know where I was. I thought they got me mixed up with another patient and put me in the wrong room. "Where were my parents?" I thought. I was scared and began to cry. Giggy, the recovery room nurse, said my parents were coming to see me. I thought to myself, "Yea! I just hope they are the right parents."

A few hours after they left, the doctor came in and said, "Hello, Bo, I am Dr. Harburg and I'm going to take you up to your room. Do not eat or drink and keep your leg straight."

I slept for a long time. The only thing I really remember was waking up that afternoon and Dr. Harburg was telling my mom that they were going to do major surgery on me. I went back to sleep.

Later that night, I woke up and a lot of people were in my room. I called my mom over to my bed. She came over and sat down. I screamed. Everybody turned their attention to me.

My mother said, "What's wrong?"

I said, "My hip! My hip!"

She said, "What about your hip?"

"You're sitting on it!"

Everyone laughed; so did I.

When we got the news about Bo's type of cancer and that his prognosis was not very good, we were, needless to say, dev-

astated. We resented every doctor who entered Bo's room because each one seemed to only want to tell us more bad news.
I have to say, in retrospect, that those doctors were amazing.
They were able to relate to us this impending nightmare and
yet did not jerk every bit of hope from us. I suppose at the time
they were quite sure that Bo's case was hopeless, but they were
still able to give us a glimmer of hope.

My first reaction to all the horrors of the side effects of
chemotherapy was "Why bother? It probably won't do him
any good anyway, and besides, what a hideous way to live —
losing one's hair, throwing up all the time, feeling sick most of
the time." The doctors reassured us that children were wonderful about it, adjusting to the situation much better than
adults, and that we would be very surprised. They even went
so far as to say that the children, as a rule, usually "carry" the
adults as opposed to the adults "carrying" the children.

I remember thinking to myself, "Yeah, well they don't
know Bo — he's a very sensitive, insecure little boy and this
will do him in. He won't be able to handle it." (I learned very
early that I had misjudged my son and that I didn't know him
as well as I thought I did. I also learned that maybe the doctors
might know what they were talking about and that, maybe, I
should listen to them a little more closely rather than resent
them.)

In the middle of that night, I woke up scared. So
we prayed about it. Then I felt better about it.
The next morning I was woken up by the
nurses. Before I was hardly awake, they gave me another
shot in the seat. I cried. My mom cried and even my dad
cried. I knew this was a dangerous operation, because I
had never seen my dad cry before.

I said, "I am scared."

My mom said, "God will take care of you."

Back then I did not trust God very much. So I was
still a little bit scared. The nurse came in to take me and
we were still scared. We all laughed and then they put me
on a stretcher. As I went out of my room, people I knew
were lined up against the wall. I waved to all of them, but
they just smiled at me.

When I woke up from the operation, I was in the same room I was in the day before. Only this time I knew where I was. I stayed there awhile and then I moved to a different room called intensive care. I spent the night there and then went back to my regular room. My stomach hurt. I was not used to stitches.

I had a lot of tubes in me. In a couple of days, they took out my nose tube. Then they took out my drain in my stomach. They were both painful.

I had a lot of people who came to see me. My grandmother, Mimi, brought me a monkey puppet that squeaked when you opened and closed its mouth.

One night my mom was talking on the phone in my hospital room. Then I heard her say, "Well, Bo is going to have to take chemotherapy." That is when I got scared!

I screamed, "Mom, get off the phone."

She hung up and said, "What's wrong?"

I was crying and I said, "I'm sorry I screamed at you."

She said, "That's okay, but what's wrong?"

"Tell me what chemotherapy is," I said.

She said, "It's when the nurse puts a needle in your vein and gives you medicine through the needle." Then she said, "It can make you sick and make you lose your hair."

"Lose my hair!" I said. "People will laugh and make fun of me if I lose my hair. Why do I have to take this medicine?"

Then she told me the real thing.

She said, "When the doctors operated on you, they found a tumor that was the size of an apple. The reason you are taking the medicine is that they think that maybe they left some cancer cells in your body and they need to kill them."

I was so mad that I said, "Cancer cells — I could catch cancer from that!!!"

Then we talked about how there were millions of different kinds of cancer. And that some people survive it and some people die from it. And I got scared at the thought of dying. But my mom said there is no reason to

be afraid because for us Christians, dying is like going to
spend the night with your best friend. She asked me who
did I like to spend the night with the most. And I said
Hunter (my cousin who lives in Austin). So my mom said
heaven would be like going to stay with Hunter, only
even better. I did not feel as afraid of dying as I did before.
Then we prayed about it. I felt better! I felt so good that I
started laughing hard.

Our telephone rang continuously during this time. I
could hear my parents tell my story over and over to
friends who cared. One phone call came from my camp
counselor from last summer. His name was William Os-
borne, and he had heard about me from the head of the
camp. My mom was talking to him on the phone and I
heard her say, "The doctors say that we need a miracle."
That scared me to death because I just knew that miracles
did not happen very often. So when my mom hung up the
phone, I called for her to come into my room. I was really
upset and told her what I had heard her say to William.
My mom answered me by saying, "Bo, do you realize that
miracles occur every day? Do you realize that every time
a baby is born it is a miracle? And do you realize that
every time the sun comes up and goes down it is a miracle? And actually the fact that our bodies exist and usually repair themselves when they are sick is a miracle.
God performs miracles every day all day long." I was relieved to hear this. Even though I knew it was true, I had
never thought of all these things as God's miracles. When
you really stop and think about it, this world is amazing.

A few days after that we went home for Christmas. A
lot of people came by and brought a lot of presents. My
brother and sisters didn't know what was going on.

**When I realized that Bo had heard me say to William that
we needed a miracle, I remember being panicked that he had
heard it and maybe sensed the urgency in my voice. On my
way to his room, I hoped that I would be able to explain my**

statement well enough so that Bo wouldn't be afraid. When the explanation of what a miracle is came out of my mouth, I was amazed. It was definitely God speaking for me, and while I said it I also listened and realized that miracles *do* actually occur every day and that we need to recognize them and be thankful. Bo was very calmed by this explanation. So was I.

There is always so much chaos at our house Christmas week that the other children weren't really aware of the extra presents people were bringing just to Bo or the extra food that was brought by people who didn't ordinarily bring us food. The children were too young to understand what was happening. Mary Kessler, our oldest, was twelve, Charlie was seven, and Alexandra, three.

When Larry and I finally had time to sit down and talk to them, we simply told them that we had a hard battle ahead of us and that there were going to be some bad times ahead for Bo, but that there would also be some good times too. We emphasized how important it was for us to stay close as a family and to talk about things as much as we could. They seemed very receptive, but I don't think they were really able to grasp what we were telling them. After all, Bo still looked like Bo, and though he was a little weak from surgery, he was getting better every day.

I also must say that that Christmas was probably the most special Christmas we had ever had. Our extended families and close friends spent a lot of time at our house during the holidays simply loving each other and caring about each other and reassessing our priorities. We didn't do the usual party circuit, where each guest feels compelled to expound on the horrors of the Christmas traffic or how terrible the sales clerks have become or other important items of conversation. A truly blessed Christmas it was in the full sense of the word.

It is unfortunate that it so often takes a crisis situation to make us stop and take the time to sense God's presence and his grace. The phrase that one hears from a very young age, "the peace that passeth all understanding," is such a powerful truth, but one can't really understand its meaning unless he has experienced that peace. Here we were facing every parent's nightmare, and yet we felt a peace and a love that we had never known. God does some truly beautiful things in this world, but we probably miss so many of them while worrying about worldly things.

In one of the daily devotional books that someone had given us, it was written: "Be thankful for your hard times as well as your easy times because it is through those hard times that you experience God's true peace."

So we, with Bo, began praising God for everything, bad as well as good, and we learned very quickly that God would carry us through anything, if we would simply allow Him to do so.

We went to church Christmas Eve and had a party afterwards. A lot of people asked how I was doing and gave me a lot of Christmas cards that said "Get Well." Christmas that year was a great Christmas. We were closer to God than we had ever been before, and we were very thankful that we were all okay that Christmas. We spent much time talking about the meaning of Christmas — about when Jesus was born and the whole Christmas story. Jesus — the Son of God.

The next week it was time to start chemotherapy. The children did not look very well, they looked strange. They did not have very much hair. The nurse fussed at my mom for being five minutes late. That day I got sick late in the afternoon. I didn't think I would get sick. We talked about how I might and probably would lose my hair. We made jokes about my possibly being bald. My mom said she thought it was great that I could laugh about it and that she hoped I'd be a good sport about it when it really did fall out. I said I didn't want to go to school, but my mom said it would be okay. And when it did start falling out it was okay. It itched a lot, but it was okay.

———

The first day that we went into the clinic was one of the worst days that I can recall. I felt this avalanche of fear coming down on me. It must have shown on my face because one of the mothers signaled me to come sit by her. She seemed so in control of her situation, and I was awed by her composure. She didn't even seem concerned that her six-year-old daughter didn't have a hair on her head. She introduced herself as Tricia and said that Kristy had been having chemotherapy for two years and seemed to be doing fine. She told me that when Kristy was first diagnosed the doctors said she probably would not survive more than a few months. This sounded very familiar. Tricia told me that she had decided then that she was not going to give up fighting this disease and that it was this attitude that had gotten her this far. She told me that the first trip to the clinic was always the worst and that someday I would feel very comfortable there.

I can't even describe the comfort this young mother gave me. I realized at this point that I, too, could handle this situation and that I was not going to give up. I also vowed to myself that I would, someday, do the same for some poor mother bringing her child into the clinic for the first time.

And there were some funny things that happened about my bald head. One thing was when we were in church one time. A little boy was sitting with his mother behind us. The little boy said loudly, "Hey Mom, look at that boy — he doesn't have any hair." The mother quickly slapped her hand over the little boy's mouth saying, "Sh-Sh!!!" The mother was real embarrassed, but I thought it was funny. My mom and I laughed.

One night not long after that Giff Nielsen called and asked if he and Alan Ashby, the Astros catcher, could come and pray over me. My mom said that that would be great. Giff and Alan are Mormons. Mormons are a different kind of Christians who believe that sometimes they have special powers of healing. They came over and Giff made a wonderful talk about how each of us has an important purpose on this earth and that we should each fulfill that purpose. He said that I had been chosen to fulfill a very important purpose and that I should follow God's word very closely in everything that I do. Right as they were going to put some oil on my head, my grandfather, who is a retired Episcopal priest, walks in my back door whistling and calling "Anybody home?" It was very funny timing because he didn't really know what was going on. My aunt Eckie and my godmother Ginger both looked at each other like "What are we going to do now?"

Aunt Eckie thought quickly and said, "Daddy, we are having a prayer; would you like to join us?"

Big Daddy said "Sure" and came in and sat down.

January 1983

I have to give a lot of credit to my sister, Eckie, and her family. Eckie helped teach all of us how to pray, especially Bo. She spent many hours talking to him about God and about how important it was to talk to God daily, not just when one needed something. She came over practically every day to visit with Bo and to pray with him. Her family also went out of their way to include Bo and the rest of our children in everything they did. The kids accepted Bo as he was, skinny and bald. It didn't seem to matter to them. They really made him feel special, and this made things a lot easier for Larry and me.

The children and the teachers at school were also incredible to Bo and to us. Before Bo went back to school in January, the teachers and staff met with all the children and explained every detail of Bo's disease including the side effects of chemotherapy, mainly the hair loss. So when Bo showed up at school sans hair, no one appeared shocked and no one stared or made any comments. (With the exception of the eighth grader who called him a "dork" because of his hat.) And after listening to other mothers in the clinic relating unfortunate incidents at their children's schools, I realized how blessed we were that River Oaks Baptist handled the situation as beautifully as they did.

 After taking chemo for a few weeks something bad happened from the chemotherapy. I had this medicine called Vincristine, which my

15

mom told me might make me very constipated. The first
week I was constipated. The second week I had the medicine was terrible. My mom had gone to lunch and I was
alone with Riri, our housekeeper for fourteen years, at our
house. Suddenly, I got a terrible cramp that would not go
away. It hurt very badly. I wish I could have been dead at
that moment, but life goes on. Riri called my mom who
told her to call Aunt Eckie. I went to sleep for a while, and
when I woke up Eckie and her Bible study friend were
standing in my room. They said a prayer for me which
was very, very nice. They asked God to help me get rid of
my cramps. I felt better after the prayer. We went outside
to look at my dog's new puppies that had been born in December.

When we got out there, we noticed one puppy was
bigger than the others and we decided to name him
Moose. After we played outside awhile, I went in because
I wasn't feeling well and was weak. They came upstairs to
say goodbye. Suddenly, I got another cramp. I jumped
around the room screaming like a wild man. My mother
came in.

She said, "Calm down."

I screamed, "I need to say a prayer." She said, "Calm
down and we will." The pain was hard to bear at the beginning of the prayer, but I was calm by the end.

Mom said it was probably constipation. The cramps
continued into the next day. We prayed so much that we
did not even concentrate to pray because it came so easy.
That night my parents were going to a hotel to get a break
from this problem. I felt I needed a break too, but I had to
live with it. We were supposed to spend the night with
our grandmother. I had cramps at her house and she
prayed with me. That night she had guests for dinner. It
was an embarrassing time because I doubled over with
pain and had to crawl out to the next room. My grandmother excused herself and came to pray with me. The
prayer came easily.

The next day my parents came to pick me up. I was
still hurting off and on. My mom and I sat in our living

room and talked. First we talked about Suzannah Sinclair (a girl who had died of a brain tumor the week I was diagnosed) and how she and her mom had had some really special times and talks when she was sick and that we would do the same. Then we talked about how Christ had suffered for us on the cross and how we should try to be like Him. Then we prayed and asked God to help us be strong and courageous. My mom also told me that she and my dad didn't have a very good night away because they worried about me. I felt that that night had been a waste for my mom and dad, and I was sorry that their break had not been better. I was still having cramps.

Then Aunt Eckie came to get me and we went to the store. I had a bad cramp and doubled over. Aunt Eckie said to me to remember how Christ had suffered for us and we know that it was harder than this and that I should maybe handle it by thinking of Christ. Thinking about it that way made it more bearable for me. Then we went to her house and we painted some tiles.

The next morning we flew on someone's plane to the Wallace's ranch. My hair continued to fall out in mounds everywhere. No one seemed to care though.

It was very cold that day. We went out on the lake in a paddle boat. While we were out on the lake I got another cramp and we prayed once again and it felt better. I was really learning how prayer could help and how God might not answer your prayer with what you necessarily want and that you sometimes have to look for the answer and not expect it to come right to you always. And if it's not the answer you want, God gives you the strength to live with His answer. And he never gives you more than you can handle. That is very important to remember.

There are a lot of things in life that could go wrong that don't, and we should thank God for those things. An example is that the plane we flew to and from the ranch on was very small and cramped, and I was very grateful that I didn't have a pain on the plane. That would have been awful.

The next morning we went into the clinic for a five-

day treatment. The doctors looked at me and saw that I
was sick and sent me home without chemo. I was happy
that I didn't have to have chemo.

That afternoon I was in so much pain that my mom
took me back to the hospital where they admitted me.
They took x-rays and drew lots of blood. I was pretty
much baldheaded at this point but I felt so bad that I
didn't really care. As it turned out, I was constipated because one of the side effects of the drug Vincristine is that
it screws up your bowels. After many enemas and three
days later I went home.

After that ordeal, I did very well. Except for my bald
head I looked and felt great — so great that my mom and
dad jokingly decided that they must have gotten my hospital records and x-rays mixed up with some other child.
We fictitiously named that "other child" Bob Neihouse.
We decided that poor ol' Bob Neihouse was really the
sick one but since they had his records mixed up with
mine, they sent him home as healthy even though he always felt bad. And here I was feeling terrific and yet they
were telling me that I had a terrible illness. We made
many references to poor ol' Bob Neihouse.

Chemotherapy became a way of life for us. Every three or
four weeks we knew that Bo would go to the clinic as an outpatient and spend several hours, or several days, getting i.v.
medicines and then go home and throw up for about a day or
two. It was an unpleasant fact, but it was bearable. Those
times that I spent with Bo were in fact almost enjoyable because he never lost his sense of humor. Even at his sickest, he
would raise his head and make some ridiculous comment
such as "Next time they give you an option of going through
this experience, let's turn it down, okay?" We would all break
up laughing and tensions would ease.

We would also pray a lot. Every prayer that Bo would say
aloud always ended with "Please put joy in our hearts." And
we did have a special kind of joy.

I went back to school between treatments still feeling great. The kids at school were all very nice to me and didn't say anything to me about my bald head. I had a lot of different and funny hats that people had given me to wear. There was a hat with red wings and another hat that looked like a bat with big black wings that spanned about two feet. I was going into one of my classes sporting that bat hat when an eighth grader said to me, "You look like a 'dork' with that hat on." I was scared of that eighth grader so I just said "Shut up" and slipped inside the door. Later I got in the car with my mom and told her the story. I told her that I had only said shut up but that I wished I had said, "You look like a 'dork' without the hat." We both cracked up laughing in the car. That story quickly went around to all my family and relatives. When the teachers heard about it they immediately wanted me to tell them who the eighth grader was, but my parents and I decided that that eighth grader probably didn't realize why I had the hat on or he wouldn't have said a word. Everyone in the school was so incredibly nice to me. They made me feel like such a hero; it was a very happy time in my life. Sometimes I felt so special that I felt a little embarrassed and I did not always know what to say. I was in a Christian school and it was very evident that the school was leading them and me in God's way.

I was surprised to find out during one of my treatments that the doctors had decided to do "second look" surgery in March (two months away). They explained to me that they needed to go in to see if there were more cancer tumors inside of me and that way they could tell if they needed to change my medicine and/or add new medicines. My family had been planning to go to Disney World for a year, and it just so happened that my surgery was scheduled one week after our trip. That was very lucky (or was it God's wonderful planning ?).

We had a wonderful trip despite the beginning, which was a little disorganized. My daddy got home only thirty minutes before we were supposed to leave. Nobody could find his shoes and everyone was having trouble getting his suitcases out to the car. My mom and dad were arguing about being so late to catch the plane. We all ran out and hopped in the car and turned on the engine. Dad said, "Does everyone have everything; do you boys have on your belts?" I answered "yes Dad" but my little brother Charlie said, "I forgot mine." Dad had to turn off the engine, unlock the door, turn off the burglar alarm, and let Charlie run up to his room to get his belt. Charlie got back in the car while Dad locked up the house again and got back in the car and started to back out again. Then my little sister, Alexandra, yelled from the back seat that she needed to go to the bathroom so we pulled back in and Dad went through the same routine while Alexandra went inside. Our yardman, Robert, was hysterical laughing at the whole scene. It was pretty funny.

We finally got on the road. We were all laughing at ourselves. We were so late by this time that my dad was gripping the steering wheel very tightly, my mom was biting her nails, and we four children were sitting very quietly wondering if we were going to make it. When we finally got to the airplane, they were literally shutting the door to the plane as we got on.

We were going first to see Ganga and Big Daddy (my mom's parents) who were staying in Beaufort, South Carolina. The plane first landed in Jacksonville, Florida, and then we went to Savannah. We then found out that our luggage had been dropped off in Jacksonville. It caught up with us three days later.

Beaufort was beautiful. We went to a daffodil farm. It was covered with acres of daffodils and the people that owned it let us pick as many daffodils as we wanted. We came home with a lot of flowers that day. We also went to Paris Island and watched the Marines march. The next day we went to a beach and had a fun picnic. I was feeling great even though the week before I had had a round of chemo. It was really good to see my grandparents; they had a neat house and were hoping to move up there. They are a lot of fun to be with.

Next we drove to Disney World. It took us a day and a half. When we got there it was pouring down rain but we were all very excited anyway. Even though the weather was not so great, we still had a wonderful time and it took our minds off of what was going to happen next week. We didn't even really think about it until the last day. The few times that I did think about it I turned it over to God and knew that He would take care of it, so then I didn't worry any more.

While we were in Disney World, waiting in lines, I would notice people staring and whispering about Bo. My maternal instincts really came out — I was ready to kill everyone for noticing. Bo either didn't notice or didn't care. He once said about his baldness, "It's everyone else's problem, not mine, because they are the ones who have to look at me." He even made jokes about his hair (or lack of) and made everyone feel very comfortable about his appearance.

He also claimed at one point that it could be to his advantage. It was when a friend of his called me and said that he was doing a report on cancer and did I think that it would bother Bo if he could ask him some questions about the treatments and tests. (This friend attended the most academically challenging school in Houston, a school which had disqualified Bo a few years prior.) I asked Bo, and he was more than happy to expound on the mysteries of chemo, CAT scans, i.v.s, etc. He even volunteered to get some of the disposable paraphernalia the next time he was at the clinic for his friend to use in his exhibit. Teasingly, I told Bo that maybe he could go to the school as a "live" exhibit. Not one to be upstaged, Bo responded without hesitation, "You bet I will — I'm sure that's the only way I'll ever get in St. John's."

I remember thinking to myself, "Boy, did that school miss out!" I'm not sure that the friend ever got the joke.

 We came home on Saturday night and checked into the hospital on Monday; surgery was scheduled for Tuesday morning. On Monday they took x-rays and drew blood and did a CAT scan. When you have a CAT scan, you have to drink a whole lot of fluid and hold it in your bladder for a real long time. When you are on the table and they are taking pictures of your stomach the only thing that hurts is your bladder because you need to go to the bathroom but they won't stop the procedure and let you go. And sometimes you just can't hold it anymore. This happened to me on the CAT scan. I urinated on myself and then I was real embarrassed. The nurse reassured me that it wasn't a big deal, that it certainly wasn't my fault, and that it happened to a lot of people. Your bladder can only hold so much at a time. I then went up and took a bath in my room. Dr. Harberg, the surgeon, came to my room and told my mom that the CAT scan looked clear, and he was real excited.

That night we got a pass to go out to dinner. We were pretty nervous but also confident that everything would go well.

The next morning the nurse came in to give me my pre-op shot. I was terrified. She finally convinced me that it wouldn't hurt that much, and she was right. I was also really afraid that the operation was going to hurt more than the first operation. When it was over it wasn't nearly as bad as the first. I guess when you expect something to be terrible and you worry about it a lot, it usually doesn't turn out to be as bad as you expected. Maybe this is God's way of helping us get through bad situations.

After the shot I began feeling drowsy and I tried to go to sleep, but they came to get me before I was really asleep. The only other thing I remember was going into the operating room and then going to sleep. When I woke up I was in the pediatric intensive care unit. When my mom came to see me, she brought my two stuffed animals, Chip and Dale (two chipmunks that I had bought at Disney World). She sang the song that I made up in Disney World about the chipmunks and made the two animals dance on my bed. It was the first thing that made me smile after my surgery. All of a sudden my heart monitor began beeping because my heart rate had gone up suddenly. The doctor told my mom not to talk to me very much because it got me too excited and I was not stable enough to get really excited.

This surgery was a lot more risky than Bo's first. The surgeon removed the entire right lobe of Bo's liver. Bo lost a lot of blood, and we didn't think he was going to make it through the night. It was probably the most frightening moment I have ever experienced in my life. I have often thought that God had considered taking Bo that night, but when He looked down at my hysteria he realized that it wasn't the right time, that He still had a lot of work to complete in me.

When the pathology report was completed, everyone was thrilled that no cancer was found. It gave Larry and me a little more hope than we had had, even though the doctors continued saying that it almost always recurs. We still enjoyed the brief moment of optimism. (There is something to be said for even false optimism.)

The next six months were relatively uneventful as far as Bo's illness was concerned. He still had chemotherapy every three or four weeks, and he was down for about a week each time but then bounced back each time. We did learn to appreciate our days a lot more, and we spent more time together as a family.

And during those times when Bo was recuperating from his chemo, we had some very special neighbors and friends who would come and simply "be" with us at our home. We will be eternally grateful for those who endured the bad times with us.

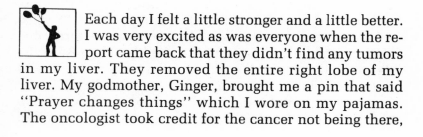 Each day I felt a little stronger and a little better. I was very excited as was everyone when the report came back that they didn't find any tumors in my liver. They removed the entire right lobe of my liver. My godmother, Ginger, brought me a pin that said "Prayer changes things" which I wore on my pajamas. The oncologist took credit for the cancer not being there,

the surgeon claimed he had gotten it all in the first surgery, but we knew who to give the credit to. Thank you God.

I healed very quickly. When we were asking the doctors when I could go home, at first they said maybe Easter Sunday, then they said maybe the Saturday before Easter because I was doing so well and I finally went home on Good Friday because I was doing so well.

We kept hearing reports of families we knew who were having a member being diagnosed as having cancer. I began thinking about it, and this theory came to my mind. God promised after the flood of Noah's Ark that he would never flood the world again but maybe cancer was going to be His way of destroying this world as we know it. It seems like everyone at some point either gets it or is close to someone who will get it.

My little brother Charlie and little sister Alexandra spent Easter weekend at my cousins' ranch so Mary Kessler, my older sister by a year, and I were the only children at home. Easter morning I was trying to decide if I felt well enough to try to make it to church. I decided that God had done so much for me in the last couple of weeks keeping me alive that I really wanted to make the effort and go to church to thank Him. So we did. And I did very well in church. I loved being there and seeing all the flowers and hearing all the music. I told God thank you for everything he had given me especially in the last few weeks.

After church we went over to my grandmother's house. My cousin, Palmer, wanted me to eat so I could gain some weight so she got a whole pack of Lifesavers and put them in my mouth all at once. After that she made me eat a lot of brownies. It was very funny. We also had an egg toss with my dad using raw eggs. He threw one from a distance and I caught the shell but the rest of the egg went all over me. It was a mess but very funny. It was a wonderful Easter.

Another funny thing that happened to me was when my camp counselor, William (the one who had called back in January), had called one Saturday and said he was coming in from Austin to see me. He said that he would be at my house at around 4:00 Saturday afternoon. That afternoon at around 3:00 my dad and I went out to rent a movie and go to the hardware store and to get a hot dog at James Coney Island. Somehow we had all forgotten that William was due at our house in only one hour. Right after we had left, my mom, still at home, remembered and was terrified that we had forgotten and would not be home when William arrived. So my mom got on the phone and called all the places that she knew we were going and told each place to look for us and to tell us to please call home immediately. And the only way she could think of to identify us was "a little boy who doesn't have any hair with his fat daddy." (Daddy really isn't all that fat, just plump.) We ran our errands and ended up at James Coney Island. When we got our hot dogs and got up to the cash register, this lady looked at us and all of a sudden said, "Phone home!!!" Dad and I looked at each other and then at her and Dad said, "What?" She then said that some lady had called looking for a fat man with his bald son and that we had to be them. We laughed and called home and then went home. William had already arrived and had been visiting with my mother. We had a nice visit. He brought me some different mineral rocks which we had studied at camp.

April 1983

One day after I had gone back to school, I noticed a note on my teacher's desk which was from a reporter from the *Houston Chronicle* that talked about doing an article on the school and how they were handling my situation. The day that they came to take pictures of my class, I was at home because I was having chemotherapy. Since I was not there, they wanted a black and white picture of me. The only black and white picture that my mom could find was one year old. I was kind of disappointed that it didn't show my bald head because that was the way I was back then, that was me. The article was about me and about a man named Rick Smith who was the chaplain at Hermann Hospital who had come to the school to help the other children understand what was happening to me and to reassure them that they could not catch cancer from me. Rick would come to our classroom once a week and visit us. He also took us on picnics and bike rides and fun things like that. We loved the article when we saw it; it was a happy article and was nicely written.

———————

Bo loved seeing his picture in the newspaper; it made him feel like a hero and a really special person. Bo had a real gift for finding and focusing on the good aspects of his disease.

26

And all this attention was definitely one of the good aspects as far as he was concerned.

Other than the nausea and vomiting and constipation, there were only two other really bad side effects from the chemotherapy. One happened one night when I was asleep. My nose started bleeding, and we couldn't get it to stop. I had had nosebleeds a lot in my life but never like this one. My dad called the doctor but by the time he finally called us back, my nosebleed had stopped; at least we thought it had stopped. When my dad woke me up to go to school, I was very weak and I began throwing up blood; and my nose started bleeding again. My dad called the doctor again, and he said for my parents to bring me into the clinic. (The clinic is at the hospital.) When we got there they drew some blood and found that my platelet count was way down. Platelets are things in your blood that cause your blood to harden so it will stop bleeding. Anyway, they sent me to the emergency room and gave me a blood transfusion. I felt better afterwards. I then went home and slept for the rest of the afternoon.

The other side effect was a backache that I would get when they would give me a drug called Actinomycin-D. The doctors said that there was no way the drug could be causing me to have back pain, so they ran some tests like x-rays and bone scans to see if there was more cancer, but they could find none. So the next month they gave me the Actinomycin-D and, again, I had the very same pain in the very same place in my back. The doctors still could not understand, but they quit giving me so much of that drug. This is when I realized that the doctors really don't know everything and that God alone is the only one who really knows everything and that we should put all of our trust in Him.

Everything was really going great that spring. I looked and felt great except for no hair. I got to go to the River Oaks tennis tournament with my class. When one

of the matches was over, I got to have my picture taken
with Ivan Lendl and to meet him. (He had just won the
match.) I spent a lot of time with my cousin, Todd, who
was also one of my best friends. It was a lot of fun.

It was time for baseball season to begin, but it hadn't
been very long since my last surgery so I couldn't play.
But my longtime coach, Mr. Perkins, let me be the bat
boy. He even got me my own shirt with my name and
"Bat Boy" on it. That was a really special shirt and really
made me feel part of the team. I did get to play in the last
two games. I don't remember how I did, but that really
didn't matter; I was just glad to get to play.

Back when Bo was first diagnosed and his prognosis was
so grim, I wondered why we were even attempting these medicines; what was the use? But we were eventually persuaded
that it might slow tumor growth and therefore buy us some
time. And time — quality time — was definitely something we
needed.

I became fairly comfortable with Bo's having the chemotherapy. It simply became part of our routine, and I was glad
that we were doing something to try and combat the disease.
Though we were told from the beginning that the drugs they
were using could be fatal, I had enough faith that the doctors
would know the limits and not exceed them. And Bo endured
the side effects with such valor and courage that he pulled us
along. As we reached each crisis, we would focus on getting to
the other side of it. We soon learned from experience the expected side effects of each drug and the length of the duration
and recovery period. Thus we would gauge our planned activities around Bo's treatments. We became adept in our calcula-
tions as his treatments continued.

The only time I really felt as if the doctors were not listening to us was when Bo's backache would occur within hours of
the administration of the drug Actinomycin-D. They continually told us that there could be no relationship between the
drug and the backache, yet it became so obvious to us. We
could practically predict to the minute when the backache

would begin. (It is my understanding that since Bo's ordeal, more patients have had the same problem with this particular drug.)

As frustrating as it was, I had to keep in mind that we are all human, including the doctors, and they were doing the best that they knew how. They were/are constantly learning and practicing new things. Perhaps this is why it is called the "practice of medicine." It hasn't been perfected yet.

May 1983

 Another exciting thing that happened to me was
Field Day at school. Field Day is a day at school
that we have a lot of different athletic events.
We don't have any classes at all, and it is a lot of fun. The
year before I had won first place out of all the third grade
classes, and it was probably the most exciting thing that I
had ever done. This year I knew that I probably wouldn't
do very well because of all my surgeries and the chemotherapy treatments making me so weak. When they
started calling out the awards, they started with the first
place first and then second place next and so on. I finally
heard my name called out for winning the sixth-place rib-
bon. I was so shocked and went up to the stage with a big
smile on my face while everyone cheered and some people even stood up while they were clapping. What a wonderful feeling that was.

One day my PE coach, Mr. O'Keefe, brought me
something in a white box. Inside there was a large trophy
that had a victory figure on top and beside the figure on
its own pedestal was a cross. Engraved on the trophy was
"Bo Neuhaus — First Place in Fight for Life." It was the
biggest trophy I had ever gotten, and I was thrilled to get
it. It really meant a lot to me.

Things continued to go along just great. I was still
having chemotherapy every three weeks, but it wasn't too
bad. Everything was so great in fact that we sorta forgot to

talk to God and spend a lot of time in prayer. I mean we went to church every Sunday and we said blessings at mealtimes and everything — but we just didn't spend a whole lot of quality time thinking about Him. One day Aunt Eckie said to me, "You know, Bo, when you are hurting or in pain we are the first to go to God for help. But now that everything seems to be okay, we hardly ever pray. We need to not only ask God for help but we also need to thank Him for each and every day that He gives us and to remember all the wonderful things that he has given us. The Lord's Prayer says to us 'Give us this day, our daily bread' — it talks about today, not tomorrow or the next day or next week, but today. It only mentions today. So we should begin each day by thanking Him for the day." And she was so right. After that, nearly every day when we were leaving for school or eating breakfast, my mom would say to us, "Have you thanked God for this day yet?" So I would and it made me feel very grateful and good.

June, July, August 1983

We spent a lot of time at the bay that summer. I swam a lot to try to keep in shape. I swam 100 laps in my grandmother's pool, and it made me feel so good even though I was tired. I also learned to sail that summer on a sunfish. That was fun, too. On the Fourth of July we always have an event at the bay called the "TCYC Olympics." (TCYC is the name of our yacht club.) We have a lot of funny relay races and games. One of the events is a pie-eating contest. I got to represent our team, and I won. I was excited to win. I was also very full. It was a really fun summer.

Sometime during the summer I received a letter from Mr. Perkins, my baseball coach, telling me that he was going to start a Boy Scout troop at River Oaks Baptist School (my school). He invited me to join the troop. I didn't really want to become a scout at first, but my parents encouraged me to do it. When we went to get my uniform, I got excited about it and was glad I had decided to do it after all.

September 1983

We began Scouts in the fall of 1983. The day after school started, we had our first meeting. My parents went to the meeting, and when we got home my mom was worried about all the responsibilities and she wasn't sure that I could handle it. I was not a particularly responsible eleven-year-old. But I told her that I would be responsible.

I was very busy with school in a new grade (fifth grade). We had three new boys in my class. And I also signed up to play soccer. I was not very enthusiastic about soccer because my coach only seemed to care about winning so he would only use the best players most of the time. (I was not one of his best players.) So I did not get to play very much but when I did, I played my hardest and did my best. I also used to go to my brother Charlie's soccer practices because my dad was coaching. One day at Charlie's practice I didn't feel like I could breathe very well, so I told my dad about it. Whatever the problem was finally it went away. It really did hurt though, and it scared me.

As far as Bo's continuation of physical activity was concerned, one of the best pieces of advice was given to us by Dr. Donald Fernbach, the head of the oncology unit. He told us from the beginning that we needed to treat Bo as normally as possible in all respects; i.e., discipline, social, sports, school, family. In the beginning, this was hard to understand. But as we continued this new way of life, we realized how right he was. Bo seemed to feel better about himself if he was treated the way the other children were treated with the same privileges as well as the same boundaries.

We were very proud of him for his participation in sports. He was obviously weakened every month from each bout of chemotherapy, but it didn't dampen his spirits. He was determined to build himself back up to the way he was before he became ill. The scouting trips also made him feel like a normal person. Each new accomplishment he made in scouting meant the world to him.

In retrospect, I realize how sad it would have been if we had not let him be "normal" and do "normal" things. And our letting him do all these things allowed us, at times, to forget about our situation.

October 1983

My mom had gone with Ganga, Big Daddy, and my aunt Eckie to Germany to visit my cousins Mishie and Anda who were there in school for a year. My dad was supposed to be leaving one morning to go on a fishing trip in North Carolina. The morning he was supposed to be leaving, I was getting dressed for school and the pain came again, so I told my dad that it was bad enough to call the doctor. When he called the doctor, the doctor told my dad to bring me in so that they could have a look at me. They sent us to x-ray and took a couple of x-rays of my chest. Then they had us wait out in the waiting room for a long time. My dad was afraid he was going to have to miss his plane, but he cared about me more. A few minutes later a doctor that we didn't know came out and asked me if I had a mole or a skin tag on my chest or my back. He looked at my chest and my back and couldn't find anything. He then left the room without telling us anything. I could tell something must be wrong.

Finally, the lady at the desk said we could go back to the clinic. When we got back to the clinic, the doctor told us that they were seeing something in the x-rays that looked suspicious and that they were going to want to do a CAT scan in the morning. In order to schedule a CAT scan at such short notice, you have to check in to the hospital the night before which means you have to sleep there. They let us go home to get our stuff for the hospital. On the way home I started crying because I didn't want my dad to have to miss his trip and to have to worry about me all the time. But my dad said that it was certainly all right and that things do work out because now he would be able to go on my first scout campout with me that weekend. And that maybe he could go on the North Carolina trip a few days late. Things do work out.

So anyway we checked into the hospital that afternoon and my dad bought me some models from the hobby shop. That night in the middle of the night my mom called home from Germany just to check on things. Actually, it was in the middle of the night in Germany but the middle of the afternoon in Houston. Charlie answered the phone and really couldn't hear too well, but he managed to tell my mom that Dad was in the hospital with me and then Charlie said to my mom, "Hey Mom, who is supposed to take me to soccer practice today?" My poor mom was real upset because she couldn't understand what was going on. Then Cindy, our babysitter (who was also my teacher), got on the phone and explained what was going on. Cindy also told my mom that there was no reason for my mom to come home because they weren't going to know anything until the next week anyway and that by then everyone would be home.

The next day we had to wait almost all day for them to do the CAT scan. They told my dad to go ahead and go on his fishing trip because they wouldn't get the results until late the next week anyway and there was no reason for him to stay home. After the CAT scan we went home, but on the way we stopped and got Charlie a model. When Alexandra saw Charlie's model, she made my dad go to the store and get her a toy.

The next Saturday morning Dad and I went to the school where we were all meeting for the campout. It was a really fun campout. It was very well organized. We went on a five-mile hike that afternoon, and that night we had a campfire. We sang songs and told stories around the campfire and then went to bed. The next morning we ate breakfast and had a chapel service. Our scoutmaster, Mr. Perkins, has a book that has a lot of Christian stories that he read to us. My dad had to leave early that day so he could get to his plane for North Carolina. We cleaned up the campsite and got ready to go home.

The next week I had a soccer game, and my mom's friend picked me up and brought me home. We won the game, but the coach didn't let me play very much. When I got home my mom was home. I was so surprised. I was glad to see her, but I was also sorry because she looked so tired and upset and I had really wanted her to have a good time. I felt like her trip had been somewhat of a waste.

The next week I got home from school to find my mom on the phone with one of the doctors. She did not seem very happy, so I kept interrupting her and asking her what was the matter. Finally, she hung up the phone and sat down by me. I could tell that I was not going to be very happy with the news.

She said, "The doctors found what may be a fungus in your lungs. They are running a test on it right now to see if indeed it is. If the test comes back negative, which would mean that it is not a fungus, then they have to assume that it is a tumor and they will have to operate as quickly as possible." I cried for a little bit but then I stopped and felt better because I had learned from experience that crying was not going to help or change anything. My mom was relieved and happy because she said she did not expect me to take the news as well as I did. I think we had been through this thing so many times that we were used to bad news and it therefore wasn't so hard to take this time. I had also learned from my second operation that the anticipation of the operation is a lot worse than the actual operation. So I really wasn't scared. Actually, to tell the truth, I was sort of excited because I knew that it would be okay and I knew I would get a lot of attention and that makes it sort of fun. I also had faith in God; He's never let me down before, and I knew this time He wouldn't let me down either. The next day when I was walking home from school, I was wondering whether or

not my mom had talked to the doctors and whether she
knew anything or not. When I got home, she was again on
the phone talking to the doctor. When she got off she told
me that I was going to have to have the operation. I was a
little upset about it even though I was also excited about
it.

Once again, Bo's faith strengthened mine. I was again terrified about his impending surgery, but he reassured me "that
God would continue to carry us" if we allowed Him.

When he said this, so sure of himself, I held him in my
arms and cried and thought to myself how blessed I was to
have this child to show me the way. I realized how Bo and I
had changed roles, temporarily; I had become the child, he,
the parent.

It was really wonderful being able to share my fears with
Bo instead of having to be strong all the time. And my fears
never seemed to shake his faith, but rather they reaffirmed his
faith.

The weekend before my surgery, Giff gave us
tickets to the Oiler game. The Oilers were having a bad season and the crowd was always
blaming the quarterback, Giff. It really made us sad to see
everyone booing our friend. After the game we went to
the locker room and waited outside. When Giff came out
he was all smiles and acted very glad to see us. He even
gave me the game ball. When we got home we saw some
of our neighbors who had been watching the game on TV.
I showed them the ball and told them that it was the very
ball that they had been watching. That was really neat.

The day before my surgery, I had a soccer game. A lot
of the better players were not there because they were on
a PE honors trip. You have to qualify to get to go on the PE
honors trip by running the 440-yard dash and have one of
the top six fastest times in the grade. I did not get a chance

to run in it because I was having chemo, so I therefore did not qualify. So we had only enough players to fill all the positions. That meant we all got to play the whole time. I really wanted to show the coach that I could play better than I did at practice. I really was mad that I hadn't gotten to play very much, so I played as hard as I could. I have never played that hard and was never as quick-footed. I was disappointed that I did not get to go on the PE honors trip, but it worked out for me since I got to play the whole soccer game. I guess that this is another example of how God makes things work out.

The next day we had to check into the hospital. We had to go through the usual routine of checking in at the admissions office, and it always takes forever and is so boring. When we finally got to our room we were really bored. I went out the door and knocked on the door. When my mom said come in, I did an imitation of one of the doctors who would be coming in at some point. Then I went out again and did another imitation of one of the nurses. And then I did the coffee cart lady that always comes around with her tray of food and drinks. My mom laughed and laughed and that made me start laughing, too. It was really funny, but more important it passed the time.

That night we had a pass to go out to dinner. We went by our house and all my family and relatives were there. My other aunt, Darrell, from Austin, gave me a stuffed furry bear whom I named "Surge" because of my surgery that I was getting ready to have. We went back to the hospital and went to sleep. In the middle of the night I woke up and was very thirsty but I wasn't supposed to have anything to drink. Since my surgery was scheduled so late for the next day my mom gave me a very tiny sip of water. Then I went back to sleep.

The next morning I woke up. There were a lot of visitors in my room. My grandmothers and my grandfather, aunts and uncles, and our friend Rick Smith were there. This was the same day that the United States was sending troops into Grenada to protect our people who were on the island from communist troops. I remember thinking to myself, "I wonder if when I wake up we'll be in a war." We had a long wait. This made me nervous and hyper. Finally, when they came to give me my pre-op shot I was not scared. I got very drowsy. Rick said a prayer for me and everyone in the room prayed for me. They came to get me and wheeled me down to the waiting room where you wait to go into the operating room. By the time that I got into the operating room, I was very sleepy. When I got into the operating room I remember that they put a cup over my mouth and told me to take a deep breath. I must have gone to sleep then, I don't remember. When I woke up again I was in the recovery room with Giggy the nurse taking care of me again. This was the third time that she took care of me after surgery. She had to tell me that I had had my operation already. I told her that my shoulder was hurting, and she told me that it was because of my operation. I spent one night in the recovery room and one night in intensive care. When I was in intensive care they would not let my parents in for a long time. They said that they had a really sick patient in the ICU and did not want the visitors to bring in extra germs. Finally, when they were going to let my mom in, the nurse told my mom that she might want to wait a little longer because they were going to start a new i.v. on me and that it might upset my mom to see it. My mom said, "Upset me? Why I could probably start one myself, he has had so many." It had been almost twenty-four hours since I had seen my parents, so I was very glad to see them. They then took me to a room.

This surgery was a lot easier because I didn't have as many tubes in me to be pulled out. I only had what is called an N.G. tube that goes into your stomach. It drains off whatever is in your stomach so that you won't get nauseated. When the doctor came in to pull it, he said, "Okay Bo, on the count of three I am going to slide the tube out. Ready one, two," and when he said "two" he pulled it out. I was very glad to have the tube out because then it meant that I could drink and eat some things. I got really thirsty, and when you have that tube in they won't let you have a thing to drink.

My dad came in to see me and I asked him what did they find when they operated. He told me that they found two tumors in my right lung. I knew that that was a bad sign because it meant that the cancer had spread, but at the time that my dad told me, I was too sleepy to care. When I finally was able to realize what he had said I still wasn't afraid because I had God on my side. And with Him — no matter what happens — everything will always be okay.

When Bo became fully alert after a couple of days, he and I discussed the fact that it is usually a bad sign when cancer finds its way into other parts of the body. In this conversation, he related to me how sure he'd become about God and heaven and that he realized that he couldn't really lose. If he lived, he'd be here with all of us and that would be great. But if he died, he'd be in even a greater place with Jesus and that, too, would be great. So either way, he wins. This was such a relief to know that he was free of fear.

Each day I got better and better. I was determined to go home sooner than they were expecting me to. The day before they said that I could go home my mom and dad brought my sisters and brother up to see me. They usually don't let young children visit in the hospital but this was a very slow Saturday on the floor and there were not very many patients on the floor. We went outside around the hospital grounds for a long walk. I was in a wheelchair. I was very excited and hyper at this little park where we stopped. I was trying to fool my parents by pretending that my wheelchair was out of control and was going to roll into the street with me in it. A lady who was sitting nearby on a bench saw me, and it scared her so much that she jumped up very quickly to save me. When she realized it was a joke, she did not look very happy. My mom and dad were not very happy either. Then we went back to my room. I was tired by the time we got there. When we got up there I had a couple of friends to visit me.

My mom asked the nurse if there was any way that I could go home that day. The doctor said that we could. So my whole family went home together. It was really an exciting event. And yet how often are we at home and just take it for granted? We don't appreciate it unless we don't have it. Coming home from the hospital can be a really exciting event. And so can other things be exciting if we learn to not take them for granted but to appreciate them each day.

Larry and I were called into the clinic to discuss changes the doctors were making in Bo's chemotherapy protocol. We were told that this type of tumor usually recurs between four and six months and that since it had taken ten months in Bo's case, the doctors had to assume that the medicines must be doing some good. But were they doing enough? It is all a big guessing game, they explained, and they felt some changes were indicated. A schedule for eight months had been set up. Bo was to be hospitalized every other month for four days and would be given a very potent drug called Cis-platinum. This drug can cause some serious side effects, some potentially lethal, and the patient needs to be monitored while the drug is being administered. It would also temporarily make him a lot sicker than any of the other drugs.

They considered this drug their best (and only) shot at beating this disease at this point. On the months that he wasn't having chemo in the hospital, he continued the outpatient treatments.

 The next few days I rested. Monday was Halloween and I went to visit my friends at school. They were amazed that I was out so soon and back at school. It had only been a week since my surgery. That night we went trick or treating. I didn't wear a costume because I was outgrowing them, but I did want to go trick or treating. So we went with my family and a lot of friends. I did just great; I don't remember having any problems. That night my dad and I stayed up late watching a movie on TV. All through the movie my dad kept trying to whistle. Everyone else was already asleep. After the movie my dad and I went to bed. The next morning my mom told me that my dad was sick and that he could not move the left side of his face. I was a little bit worried and asked if it was going to get better. My mom said yes but that we needed to keep all pressure off of him for a few weeks. He had something called Bell's Palsy which paralyzes the whole side of your face but usually will get better on its own. Dad was better in a few weeks, but he was sure funny looking those first couple of weeks.

I had missed a lot of scouting things that winter because of my surgery and the chemotherapy. But now I was going to be able to go on some more of the campouts. On the next one we were going to the Aransas Pass Wildlife Refuge. My dad and I were so late getting to the school to join the troop that we thought we were going to be left behind. We barely made it. We saw a lot of animals that weekend that you don't see very much because they are almost extinct. We saw some whooping cranes and javelinas. We went on hikes and played on the beach.

December 1983

One day before Christmas my cousin Todd and I decided to go to the Galleria (a large shopping mall with an ice skating rink) to go Christmas shopping for our families. First, though, I had to go get a blood count at the hospital. After they poked my finger we left because we were in a hurry to get to the Galleria; we didn't wait around for the report. My mom dropped us off at the Galleria and told us to take the bus home because there was so much traffic. When my mom got home she got a phone call from the nurse at the clinic telling her that my counts were very low and that I needed to be kept at home away from large crowds of people or I might get sick. My mom had no choice but to wait for us to get home because there was no way to find us. When we got through shopping we went to catch the bus. Todd had bought a magic set while we were shopping and decided to open it on the bus. All the people on the bus wanted to see us do the magic tricks, so we went to the front of the bus and did some tricks. Every time we did one they would all laugh and cheer. It was really funny. Todd and I really laughed, especially when we got home and my mom told me what the nurse had said. Here I was supposed to be in isolation and I was, instead, riding on a public bus doing magic tricks. We had so much fun that we wanted to do the same thing the next day, but then my mom reminded me of the bad news about my blood count.

That was another fun Christmas. I got a neat tent to use on my scouting campouts. I slept in the tent in my room Christmas night. All four of us kids slept in it. It was a little crowded, but it was fun. Another thing that I got was a remote control jeep. Charlie got one just like mine. They were really neat because they could go over things and go real fast just like a real jeep. You didn't have to have a flat surface for them to run.

It was extremely cold that winter; the lowest it got was about ten degrees, and that temperature lasted for about a week. Everyone was having busted pipes and power and water shortages. We weren't used to this kind of weather. Since it was too cold to go outside, Charlie and I sat inside with our remote controls and guided our jeeps that were outside. We would have them running up and down the sidewalks, and when cars drove by they would stop and look and wonder. They couldn't see us inside running the jeeps; all they could see were these two miniature jeeps going down the sidewalks. We also had them chase people who were walking by. It was great fun.

My chemotherapy schedule had changed since my lung surgery. They were giving me new medicines at different times. Every four weeks we had to go into the hospital and stay a couple of nights to have a new drug called Cis-platinum. It was terrible; I was up all night throwing up for a few days. It really made me feel terrible the whole time. It's a very potent drug, and they felt that this was our only chance to beat this thing. I had to do it once a month. They tried giving me a drug called Reglan, which was supposed to help counteract the nausea, but it gave me uncontrollable muscle spasms so they had to quit giving me as much. When I got home I was so weak that I could hardly walk or do anything for several days. After a few days I did feel better; in fact, I felt great.

January 1984

Between my in-the-hospital treatments I had to have outpatient treatments at the clinic. One time during one of our cold weather periods I had to go to the clinic for a long drip of medicine. These can sometimes take hours and hours. This particular drip did take a long time. The clinic was very crowded that day, and there were few places to lie down. The nurse did find me a place in a back hall to lie down on a stretcher. The hall was between two doorways that opened onto the outside where it was eighteen degrees. People kept coming in through those doors, and every time the doors opened a blast of cold air would come in. It was so cold that they kept putting blankets on me. My mom and dad were both there with me, and they were furious that the facility was so bad. I heard my dad talking to one of the doctors saying that it was ridiculous that in a city of this size and in one of the top medical centers in the world that this should be allowed. The waiting room in the front was always very crowded. The sad thing about it was that at least I could lie down this time. Everyone else taking medicine had to sit up on a bench because there was no place to lie down. And it is no fun to be sick and have to sit up at the same time. At that time my mom and dad decided that they were going to accomplish two things: they were going to fix me and they were going to fix the clinic. They were very determined.

Texas Children's Hospital is, indeed, one of the finest pediatric cancer hospitals in the country in regard to quality care. However, the facility available for the care of hundreds of gravely ill children was originally a residence building for the hospital residents back in the 1950s. The building was remodeled years ago to make space available for the Research Hematology Department. Because the department is outside of the main hospital building and possibly because seeing a bunch of baldheaded kids with i.v.'s in their arms is not a pleasant sight, this department seems to be forgotten by the hospital administration.

Bo did receive chemotherapy in exactly the conditions he described. Since his death, we were able to make available one 18x18-foot room for the children to receive treatment, rather than having to sit on the steps and in the back hall. This room was made available through the efforts of the merchants of the Carillon Shopping Center in Houston and our friends and family. We were thrilled that the hospital chose to dedicate this room in Bo's memory as he would be glad to know that kids no longer have to lie in the back hall to receive their medicines. It took us close to two years to obtain the use of this room for these children. We are still adamant that while this one room is a vast improvement, it is ridiculous to have children who are fighting for their lives and parents who are many times walking a path of financial and emotional disaster to have to spend so much of their lives in the conditions as they exist.

We are now working to improve the "creature" comforts for the patients, parents, and doctors in the clinic. Thanks to the Children's Charity Fund, a group dedicated to benefitting children who are disadvantaged, we are acquiring a computer for the clinic to improve their patient record retrieval which will aid in improving their ability to find diagnoses more quickly, correlate records, and deal with patient problems resulting from chemotherapy treatments instantaneously.

Of course, our long-term goal is the same as that of the doctors: to eliminate the need for any families to endure the experience of battling cancer and related diseases. We have a long way to go, but any contribution we can make as laymen wanting to help, we feel, is well worth the effort.

I was able to go on most of the scout campouts because my new schedule of chemotherapy seemed to work out in between times. Sometimes during the winter months my mom would think that it was too cold for me to go and I would argue with her; I usually won.

One day I was sitting in the den watching TV when Aunt Eckie came in with a lady from Germany. She introduced me to her. Her name was Julianne, and she had come all the way from Europe to pray for me. She told me of all the people in the world that were praying for me every day. There were people from Germany, Austria, and even a convent in Ireland. I really was amazed that that many people cared about me. It made me feel like I was living in a loving world. It reassured me that God really cares about me, and it made me feel good. Each day that Julianne was here we had a little prayer ceremony. While she was here several small but very real miracles occurred. (Or as my mom calls them, "God's calling cards," letting you know that He is with you.)

One happened when Julianne really wanted me to go with her to this lady's house to pray with her. This lady whom we called Mom Vivian had a prayer room. Eckie and Julianne were in the car coming home from somewhere when Julianne said, "We should go to Mom Vivian's house right now."

Eckie said, "Fine, but I am not sure how to get to her house. I know the name of her street, but I am not sure how to get to it." And just as Eckie said it, she looked up and there was a street sign with the name of the street on it. Eckie and Julianne couldn't believe it.

They came right over to get me and tell me about it and to get me to go with them to Mom Vivian's house. We went by Eckie's house to get their jackets, and as Eckie was standing on her brick steps looking down, something caught her eye. She said, "Oh my gosh, you won't believe this, come here." So I walked over to where she was standing and looked down, and there engraved on the brick as clear as anything was my name "BO." I couldn't believe it. Neither could Julianne and Eckie. Eckie's family had lived in that house for about ten years and we had never noticed that brick. Another of God's calling cards?

We then went over to Mom Vivian's house. She lived in a regular townhouse with a lot of rooms and pictures. We went and had a little prayer service, and she prayed for the people all over the world who were praying for me. After the prayer service she gave me a sheepskin rug to keep in my room to use for praying. It was a neat soft rug, and I was glad to get to use it.

Then we went over to get my cousins at school and to go to their basketball game. After that I went home with them to eat dinner with them and stayed there for a little while. It had been a very special day for me, and I was very tired when I finally went home.

The next day was the day that Julianne was leaving. So before she left we had a very special prayer service. My mom and I each held a candle and she said a beautiful prayer not asking God to heal me, but instead, thanking God for healing me. For she truly believed that I was healed.

February 1984

Aunt Eckie was scheduled to go into the hospital and have a hysterectomy. I gave her my cross to wear because she had given it to me when I first got sick and I always wore it. It was a very special cross to me, and I knew it would probably help her through her surgery. It did. She had a very easy time, and we were all very thankful.

March 1984

March was a great month for us. First of all, after watching the Olympics in February, especially the speed skaters, it made all of us want to go skate. Charlie's birthday was March 4, and he decided to have a huge skating party. It was a blast. I was so glad that I felt well enough to go. We skated really fast the whole time.

A few weeks after that it was spring break. We had planned to go skiing if the monthly x-rays of my lungs were normal — and they were!! We had always wanted to go skiing as a family, but my mom and dad always said that it was too expensive and that we couldn't afford it. But because of my illness, my parents realized that we might not have a lot of time to do all the things in life that we want to do. We learned that you shouldn't put off doing what you want or should do because you never know what might happen tomorrow to any of us. So we then figured that we could afford it.

We were really excited about going on this ski trip, but I was afraid that it might be a little bit cold. My parents and my friends who had been skiing assured me that it wouldn't be too cold. When we got out of school my mom told us that we were going to get to go two days earlier than planned because my mom's high school friend, Marilou, and her husband live in Denver and we were going to go visit them before we went to Vail. The day we were to leave, we went to the airport and found that some of our friends were going on the same plane that we were. That made the plane trip a lot of fun.

When we arrived, our Denver friends were there to pick us up, so we said goodbye to our Houston friends. We were so excited because there was snow on the ground. We jumped out of the car and started throwing snowballs at each other. My parents didn't, just us kids. The next morning we went to the Children's Museum of Denver. It was a neat place for kids, and there were a lot of fun things to do. My favorite thing about it was a room full of plastic balls waist-high that we could run around in and bury ourselves in them. After that we went to a great Mexican restaurant where there were jugglers, magicians, and puppet shows. After we finished lunch, we went back to our friends' house to get our luggage and go back to the airport to meet our skiing friends, the Perrins.

We met up with them and piled in their Suburban and traveled to Vail. That was so exciting because when we got to Vail there was so much more snow than there had been in Denver. We were a lot higher up in the mountains. The next day we went over to the slopes. Our family was very excited since we had never been skiing before. We rented skis at the slopes and got our lift tickets and got signed up for ski school. We had a ball that week, and it was so beautiful to see all of God's nature. The last day we skied so well that we skied down a double black diamond slope that the experts ski down. (Double black diamond slopes are the most difficult.) We took my dad up one of the black slopes and his skis were so big that he kept falling over the moguls and couldn't keep up with us. He got really mad, but Charlie and I thought it was funny. (He wasn't really mad; actually, he thought it was funny too.) We went on a sleigh ride that night with a lot of people from Houston. There were lots of Mary Kessler's friends from school there also. They took us to a small cabin and gave us some hot apple cider and told us about Vail in the olden days. It was a really fun trip. The friends that we stayed with, the Perrins, we didn't know that well when we first went on the trip but we really got to know them and love them while we were there. They are a family like ours who have a really good time together.

The week after we got home my mom went into the hospital to have a hysterectomy. The same week I was supposed to go on a rafting trip down the Rio Grande River on another PE honors trip. I didn't ever get a chance to run the 440 to qualify, but my PE coach said that he had never seen anyone fight cancer like I had and that anyone that could fight something so hard deserved to go. So I got to go. My dad spent the week helping me pack. We then went to the hospital to visit my mom on the way to catch my train. I was very thankful to see that my mom was okay before I left on my trip. When we got to the train station I saw all my friends, and I started to get a little homesick and nervous because I was the only one who hadn't had to qualify. I thought they probably all knew that and might make fun of me. (My physical stamina and ability wasn't what it used to be, by any means.) And I knew if I told them what Mr. O'Keefe had said to me about fighting cancer that they would all think I was just bragging. Fortunately, nobody asked any questions. I have always been a little sensitive about being away from home, so that night on the train I cried just a little bit until I got used to everything and everybody. I prayed that everything would be okay with my mom and with my trip. And it was okay.

The first thing that we did when we got there was to get on a bus and travel for about eight hours. We were way out in a desert and when we were about two hours away from the river that we were going to raft, the bus broke down. Some people thought we were going to be camping there for the night, but we got the bus fixed and got back on the road. We finally got to the river and we all jumped in and swam to the other side. The other side was Mexico, and we thought that was real neat to be able to be in either country. Then we had to cook our dinner because it was getting dark pretty quickly. There were five groups of us but we only had three backpacking stoves. Our group didn't get a stove, so I got worried that we weren't going to get to eat and I went off by myself and cried a little bit again. One reason I was sad was that I knew that my parents would want me to eat. I was always very thin because each month I would lose weight when I had chemotherapy and spend the rest of the month trying to gain it back. Anyway, Mr. O'Keefe gave me some of his water to mix with my dehydrated food and I had that for dinner. I felt better after that. We then went to bed under the stars. It was really great being out in the open, not in a tent or anything.

The next day we had a little problem. The desert that we were on was government property and our instructors warned us not to pollute or litter because they would lose their permit and we then wouldn't be able to go on the river. They discovered that in one of the groups there was a lot of trash that the group had tried to bury in the sand. They told us to take off our lifejackets because no one was going to get to go rafting because of that one group. I was very disappointed. Then the instructor said that he was going to let everyone except that one group go rafting, so we got our lifejackets back on and put our rafts in the water and got on the river. We had a blast. We had water fights and we swam a lot because it got so hot in the sun. We were still in the middle of the desert. When we stopped for lunch, the other group showed up in a raft. They got to go rafting after all, but they didn't get to do the water fights and the swimming that we got to do.

The rest of that day was the same and a lot of fun. When we stopped at sundown, we got to camp out on the Mexican side. We were in a deep canyon. This time we all were very careful to keep our campsites really clean. The instructors were very pleased at how we kept the campsite so clean. That night I was looking across the canyon and I saw a cross that looked like it was engraved into the canyon. I started taking pictures of it because it was so beautiful. I felt like God was saying hello to me.

The next day we rafted all morning until we got to the takeout point. This day it was too cold to have water fights. When we got to the takeout point, we had to then ride the bus for eight more hours to catch the 10:00 P.M. train back to Houston. We had dinner in Alpine, Texas, at the Pizza Hut. Some people had lost their money, so we all had to share. The same group that had littered in the desert turned their pizzas over on the table and made a huge mess.

One of the girls that had been on my raft apparently had the chicken pox but nobody knew it, not even the girl until she broke out in spots. (Cancer patients have to be very careful not to catch chicken pox while they are having chemotherapy; it can be very dangerous and some have even died from it.)

When we got to the train station the train was a little bit late, so we all used a pay phone to call home to see how everything was. When I called home, I was happy to know that my mom was home from the hospital. I even got to talk to her. We all finally boarded the train. We were excited about getting home the next day. We went to the snack bar to get a Coke. Somehow I forgot to pay for my Coke and the man got sorta mad until he realized that it was an honest mistake. I paid and then went back to my seat and went to sleep. When I woke up we were in San Antonio. When we finally arrived back in Houston, I was happy to see my dad and Charlie waiting for me at the train station.

When I told my dad about the girl with chicken pox, he called the doctor to tell him that I had been exposed. They had me skip chemotherapy that next week because they didn't want my immunities to be down if I happened to catch chicken pox in the next couple of weeks. I was glad to skip chemo that week.

We spent a fun Easter at the bay. Big Daddy, my grandfather, had a communion service in front of the yacht club. It was a wonderful service, and there were a lot of people there. It was a beautiful morning and great to be in the outdoors. After the service we hunted Easter eggs. It was truly a wonderful way to celebrate the resurrection of Christ.

When we told the clinic about Bo's exposure to the chicken pox, they warned us that it is very dangerous, sometimes even fatal, for cancer patients to contract chicken pox. The reason for the danger is because the chemotherapy drugs knock down the immune system, and thus lower one's resistance to infection. If a chemotherapy patient does get chicken pox, he almost always has twice as severe a case as a normal person.

I have to admit, though, I was not really worried that Bo would get chicken pox. He had been exposed on numerous occasions — even by his three siblings — and had never gotten the virus. In general, Bo had been the healthiest child in the family; that is, he rarely had colds, ear infections, or any other childhood ailments. We were fortunate from the very beginning that Bo's white blood counts (immune system) never hit a dangerous low. Many children are required to stay in isolation in the hospital for weeks at a time.

May 1984

May was not a particularly exciting month except for one thing. There was a planned scout campout in San Marcos that I was not going to be able to go to because of my chemo schedule. But since my chemo had been postponed for a couple of weeks, it worked out that I could go, and I was happy about that. We went canoeing down a river and about halfway down the river we lowered our canoes down this dam. We stopped for lunch, and after lunch we climbed up the dam and started jumping down the dam into the water. Our scoutmaster got mad because we weren't supposed to be doing it, and he thought we had been told, but I sure didn't remember being told. The fathers were even doing it. Anyway, at a later meeting we had a big commotion about whether or not we had been told.

Baseball wasn't a very good season, because I wasn't really into baseball. I was glad when school finally got out the end of May. I always looked forward to summer.

June 1984

The next few months became probably our most special months, and there was a very good reason for it.

The day after my sister, Alexandra's, fifth birthday, I was supposed to have two days of chemo on Monday and Tuesday. I went to have the routine x-rays that I had each month. After they took the x-rays, but before they got the results of the x-rays, the doctor came in to talk to my mom and me. He said that since I was doing so well they were planning to take me off chemo in a month. He did suggest that we do one more round of the Cis-platinum in the hospital in July, just to give me one last big blast. He said it wasn't necessary though he thought it wouldn't hurt anything and it might just make sure that all the bad cells were gone. But he said it was our decision. My mom said that whatever he thought was best was what we would do.

On the way home my mom and I were really excited that this whole ordeal might at long last be over. My mom said that if everything turned out to be okay, that on July 16, we would have the biggest birthday party for me that anyone has ever seen. Boy were we excited!!!

That afternoon I felt fine; the drug that I had had wasn't one that ever made me sick. Sailing camp at the bay started the next day, and Charlie and I were supposed to go to it; but since I had chemo the day that it started, I was going to be a day late. We decided to go to the bay that night (Monday), spend the night, leave Charlie there the next morning, and then come back to town for my chemo. Dad was going to come down after work.

I went out to feed the dogs right before we were going to leave, when I saw my dad drive up. I thought he was simply coming home early so that he could ride to the bay with us. When I got back from feeding my dogs, my parents asked me to come talk to them. I asked my mom if they had called from the clinic and my mom said that they had called my dad. I knew that they must have found something on the x-rays, so I burst into tears. I was right: it was in my lungs again. Then we called everyone into the room and we said a prayer and talked about it. We prayed that we would learn to live with it and not fall apart and to still enjoy life. Then my grandmother, Mimi, came by and we sat and talked. She said that she knew that I could fight whatever came to me. We then decided to go to the bay and have a good time.

I will never forget the look on Larry's face when he came home that afternoon. His face was ashen and his eyes were red. When he told me what Dr. Mahoney had said, I was astounded, and yet, I am not sure that I ever felt totally confident, in Bo's lifetime, that he had beaten the disease. Larry did give me encouragement by saying that the initial shock was the worst part, that once again, we would adjust and proceed with our lives. And he was right. We all cried together for a few minutes, prayed for guidance, and left for the bay.

I reminded Bo that we had been at crisis points before and had endured them, and we would do it again — as many times as required of us. We would make the best of them, and that is exactly what we did.

We had learned to put out of our minds the thoughts of what might happen and simply enjoy the present moments. This is how we should learn to live each day, whether or not we are in crisis.

When we got to the bay, Charlie and I got on our sailboats and sailed around while everyone else watched from the pier. We had a really fun time, but I was also very scared. Then I decided that the best thing to do was to forget about it for a while, so that is exactly what I did. I think that everyone else was scared, too. When we finished sailing, we sat on the pier talking with my grandparents, Ganga and Big Daddy, who had stopped by. We were talking about how death could happen to any of us at any time and there was no way to know when God would call one of His children home, and therefore there was no reason to sit around and wonder who would be next. That made someone think of the joke about two Christians who were sitting around talking and wondering what heaven was going to be like. They were both big baseball fans, and they were hoping that there would be baseball in heaven. They decided to make an agreement: whoever died first and went to heaven would somehow figure out a way to let the other one know whether or not there was baseball. So finally one of them died and went up to heaven. Remembering their agreement, he signaled his friend on earth and said, "I have good news and I have bad news. The good news is, there is baseball in heaven, but the bad news is, you are scheduled to pitch next week."

We laughed about it and I said to Big Daddy, "Hey Big Daddy, I hear you are scheduled to pitch next week." We all laughed again; it was a special time for us. God gives relief through laughter which helps you get through the bad times. We had a terrific time that night.

The next morning we left Charlie at the bay for sailing clinic and came back to town. I was scheduled to have a CAT scan that morning. We went to the waiting room as usual and waited for a while. A black lady whose name was Ernestine came and asked for me. I was very nervous and Ernestine could tell, so she started making jokes and being very funny with me. We were all laughing at her; she was one of the funniest people that I've ever known. And she made us all relax. I drank the awful drink that they make you drink, and then they took me in for the CAT scan. The nurses were very nice but the technician, a man, was not. My mom asked if she could stay in with me, and the man said that she couldn't.

"But I always have in the past," my mom said. (CAT scans do not hurt at all; but it is just nice to have someone you know in there with you.)

The man then replied, "It's time that your son were weaned from you."

The nurses all looked at my mom as if to say, "Don't take that from him, he's a jerk!"

So my mom said, "I don't care what you think, I am staying in here with him." Then the man started telling my mom that he knew how she felt because his eighty-five-year-old father was also very ill in the hospital. My mom then just sort of rolled her eyes. When he left the room, the nurses cheered my mom on.

Anyway, my mom stayed in the room with me and we got through with the CAT scan. My godmother, Ginger, was waiting outside the room for us. She got to meet Ernestine, too. We all went back to our house.

The next day I went back to the hospital to have a liver and bone scan. My other aunt, Darrell, came in from Austin to be with us. Our friend Elizabeth Sinclair also came up to the hospital to be with us. She gave my mom and sisters a Bible verse about how to not be afraid. She read to them Psalm 3:3–5 which says, "But you, O Lord, are always my shield from danger; you give me victory and restore my courage. I call to the Lord for help and from his sacred hill He answers me. I lie down and sleep, and all night long the Lord protects me."

After we got through at the hospital, my grandmother, Ganga, Eckie, Darrell, and my mom and I drove back down to the bay to drop me off at sailing clinic. On the way down my mom was telling me about the verse that Mrs. Sinclair had given her and how encouraged she felt after listening to it. I asked my mom what verse it was and she told me. I then told her that the night before I couldn't sleep because I was afraid of what was going to happen, so I got out my pocket Bible that Aunt Eckie had given me. (It is a small Bible, and I keep it in my duffle bag for when I am away from home; it doesn't have all of the Bible in it, just a lot of special verses.)

"What is amazing," I told my mom, aunts and grandmother, "is that Psalm 3:3–5 is exactly what I came to when I opened up my Bible." I then pulled it out of my duffle bag and showed them where I had marked it and saved the place. God obviously meant for us to see that particular verse. It gave me a great peace to know that God was still in there taking care of me and wanting me to know that He was there. I then knew that I could handle whatever was in store for me.

I was really amazed that Bo, on his own, really used the little Bible and that he kept it in his duffle bag at all times. This was the first I knew of it, and I was very impressed. I also couldn't believe that when I told him about Elizabeth's verse that he not only knew of it, but had it right there in hand. Each happening like this made me even more aware that God was most assuredly in control of our situation.

It also took a burden off of me to know that Bo really looked and depended upon God for His assurance rather than totally depending on Larry and me.

We then all talked about how blessed we were to have our faith in God and what do people who don't have that faith do when they are in a scary situation like mine. Then they dropped me off at the bay. I was glad to see Charlie, and he was glad I was back at camp.

I stayed there for the rest of the week and had a great time. I thought that I would probably be having another lung surgery the next week, but I wasn't afraid. I had done it too many times already to be afraid.

The next weekend my mom told me that they suspected that there was a tumor not only in the lungs but in the liver again as well and that the next week they were going to do what was called a "liver biopsy" to see if what they were seeing in the liver was indeed a tumor. She told me that they would deaden my stomach and then stick a long needle all the way into my liver and remove some of the tissue and then see if it was a tumor. I was afraid of the liver biopsy. It sounded like it would hurt even if they did deaden my stomach. So the next few nights I had a hard time sleeping from worrying about it. I prayed to God and it made me feel better, but I was still afraid a little bit.

As it turned out, it wasn't as bad as I thought it was going to be. But the doctor scared me because he called my parents in to show them what he had found on the CAT scan last week. We got to go home after we were through, but we didn't know the results. All that they could tell us was that we would definitely be taking another schedule of chemo.

Thus began our real test. It was confirmed that the tumors were not only in his lungs again, but back in his liver as well, making surgery no longer a viable solution. My overall reaction was not what I would have expected. I was a little bit relieved that Bo wouldn't have to endure another painful surgery again only to have this scenario repeated again in a few months. I believe that we had all grown so much spiritually that we knew that God would get us through this, just as he had gotten us through the other tough times we had experienced during Bo's illness. Had this been the situation when Bo was first diagnosed, I imagine that we would have fallen apart but as it was, we seemed to accept it and set our sites on making the best of it.

My sister Eckie, who is Charlie's godmother, sent a letter to Charlie when she heard about Bo. To me, it is a wonderful explanation to God's plan and how we have to believe that his overall plan is perfect though it doesn't always seem like it at the time. The letter reads:

Dear Charlie,

I just got a letter from Mary Kessler. She is having so much fun at camp.

I thought that while I need to write her back, I really need to write my Godchild, whom I love and miss a lot!

I hear that you went to Astroworld [an amusement park] on Monday but you told Ali [little sister] that you were going shopping instead. How funny! She would have been so miserable at Astroworld after the first thirty minutes, and yet there's no way she could understand that.

I guess it's sort of like God's plan with us. Sometimes there are things that we just can't understand, because we are like little children to God. He knows what is best and his plan is perfect, although His plan is real different from our plan sometimes. Just like if you let Ali decide to run the family. She'd probably cook Twinkies and ice cream for every meal and never clean the house or do homework or anything. Can you imagine what the place would be like in a month? Nothing against Ali, of course; she'd do a lot better than most kids her age, I'm sure. But it's so lucky that you have a Mom and Dad around to make the big decisions and keep everybody in line. A grown up mind can see a lot further than a child's mind, and God's mind can see a lot further than a grown up's mind. So we just have to put our faith in our Lord and leave the driving to Him.

The neat thing about God though is He can be your very best friend if you get to know Him. Whereas sometimes you can't reach or talk to your Mom or Dad, YOU CAN ALWAYS talk to Jesus. And the more you call Him, the easier it is to talk to Him. But you need to call Him a lot, not just when you need Him. Call Him to tell Him it's a great day or thank Him for that ice cream cone or whatever.

Anyway, I love and miss you a lot.

Love, Aunt Eckie

And to take this idea one step further, I believe that God

really hurts when we hurt. Just like when we as parents have to discipline our children. It hurts us to hear them cry as a result of that discipline, but we also know that it will be okay in the long run. And that discipline is a necessary part of growth in our children.

Bo and I began many more discussions about death and heaven. I told him that I truly believed that some day we will all be in heaven together and we will look back on his illness and realize how we were tiny little specks in God's overall plan. And though all of this seemed so important and terrible at the time, we will finally realize that we had nothing to worry about. That our eternal life is what really counts.

 When we got the results, it was very bad news. They found more tumors in my liver and there was no way that they could get it out by operating, so that there was no reason to try to remove the ones from my lungs and put me through another operation. We thought we were in trouble, but then we remembered that God was on our side and that He would take care of us, whatever the final outcome was. It really made us feel like everything was going to be okay. We knew that it was really in God's hands now and He would fulfill His will. I was still going to have to take chemo though to maybe slow it down. I was glad that I was still going to have chemo because I felt like we were not giving up on my being healed.

One day when I felt a little afraid, I asked my mom if they were just going to sit back and watch me die and my mom answered, "Of course not!" That instead they were going to sit back and watch me live just like anyone else. That gave me a lot of encouragement.

Mary Kessler left for camp for seven weeks. When I said goodbye to her I was secretly hoping that it wouldn't be the last time I ever saw her; I didn't know if I would be alive in seven weeks. I think that she was sort of afraid too, but she didn't say so.

I was supposed to be going on a Boy Scout trip to the

Smoky Mountains in Tennessee that I had been counting on all year. It was to be for ten days at the end of June. There was no way that I could go with my new chemo schedule, so I was going to have to miss the trip. My parents planned a trip to Washington, D.C. instead. I have always been a big fan of George Bush, our vice-president, and I have always wanted to see where he worked and everything.

When people that we knew heard we were planning this trip, they started making a lot of incredible arrangements for our trip. My grandmother, Mimi, called George Bush's office in Houston and arranged for us to have a private tour of the White House and some other neat things. People really cared and wanted it to be a wonderful trip for us. And it was wonderful!

July 1984

My dad, mom, Charlie, and I flew to Washington, D.C. on July 4th. We stayed in a suite at the L'Enfant Plaza hotel. The suite was given to us for the weekend by the people at Transco, a company in Houston. It was huge. It had a lot of glass, and we could see a lot of Washington from it. We could see the airport very clearly, and it was fun to watch the planes land.

That afternoon we went to the mall to see the Beach Boy concert. It was very hot and crowded; there were 500,000 people there. But it was really exciting to see it all and to see all the people. That night we got to go to the White House and watch the fireworks on the White House lawn. Only a few people were invited to watch the fireworks on the lawn, so that was exciting. The fireworks were unbelievable. The "President's Own" band was playing on the White House porch. (They were part of the Marine Corps band.) It was a wonderful evening. We walked home from the White House. We were walking against the crowds of people, and it made it difficult. The cars were just stuck in the street; they couldn't move because of the crowds of people. There were a lot of drunk people and a lot of people sleeping on benches on the mall and everything. Charlie was afraid that someone might hurt us. I was not afraid because I knew that God was with us.

The next day we had to get up really early to go on a

VIP tour of the White House. We went in a special gate and were given special passes. It was just the four of us on this special tour. We first got to see George Bush's office and go into it and look at all the things in it. We also got to sit in his chair at his desk. Next we got to see all the cabinet rooms and a lot of other rooms where no tourists are allowed to go. Then we got to see the president's oval office; we didn't get to go in it but we got to look in it. We then joined a larger group and toured the rest of the White House like normal tourists. We were so spoiled by this time that we didn't like going on the tours like regular people; we wanted our own special tour again. When we left the White House they gave us some souvenir pens and things. We then went across the street to the executive office building where the news media meets and sets up events. We saw George Bush's other office, too, and they gave us some pictures of him that the press uses a lot. This was a wonderful experience.

That night we had room service in our room for dinner because we were so tired. It started to rain and became the biggest thunderstorm that we had ever seen. We watched the planes land at the airport until the storm got so bad that the planes couldn't land anymore. We talked about how God let most of the planes land in just the nick of time before the storm hit. We played games that night and watched the storm and had a wonderful time.

The next morning we had another special tour of the FBI building. It was fascinating. They showed us a lot of things about how they catch criminals and about guns. They gave an exhibition of the shooting range. We watched with a lot of other people, but when it was over they let the four of us go behind the protective glass and see close up what they were shooting. Then we got to see the gun vault where they kept a lot of guns. They took a picture of us and said that they would mail us one.

The next day a driver from the parks department came and took us all around Washington. We went to Arlington National Cemetery and we saw the Washington Monument. We saw the Jefferson Memorial and the Lincoln Memorial. We never had to wait in a single line. There were thousands of people everywhere waiting in long lines, and our driver just marched us up to the front of every line. We felt sort of guilty, but it sure made it fun.

That night we got to go watch the Marine parade which is held outside in a beautiful courtyard. It was really interesting to watch and very impressive. It was very colorful. When it was over we went across the street to a restaurant for dinner. It was not in a very nice part of town, and there were not very many taxis. But it was amazing; as soon as we were through and walked outside the restaurant there appeared a taxi — and it was empty. And as soon as we got back to our hotel rooms we looked outside and it was pouring down rain. It became another incredible storm. We couldn't believe that the weather had held up for us so well. God wanted this to be a special and perfect trip, and so far it was.

The next day we hired a driver to take us to all the places that we hadn't seen. He came in a big bright black limousine, and Charlie and I couldn't believe it. He was so nice and knew a lot about Washington. He took us to Mount Vernon and to the National Cathedral. We also saw the Archives building and the Senate. We had him take us to a friend's house who is a congressman from Houston. We visited with them for a while at their house.

Sunday, our final day, was a perfect ending. We went to the tidal basin and rode in paddle boats. It was a gorgeous day. The weather was perfect for riding around in the little boats. When we finished the boats, we played in a nearby park. While we were there the presidential helicopter flew over our heads. It had just taken President and Mrs. Reagan back to the White House after their weekend away. That was exciting to see, but we wished we had been at the White House to see it land. We checked out of our hotel and went to the airport and flew home.

We really couldn't believe how perfect the trip had been; everything had gone like clockwork. It was as if God Himself had planned the whole trip to show us how well

He does plan and to make us realize that His overall plan
is perfect also. Sometimes, it is hard to believe that His
plan is perfect because things (my cancer) might not be
going as we would have had them, but somehow they always work out.

**We were fortunate to be able to take these special trips.
They allowed us to spend quality time alone with each other
and helped us to put out of our minds the gravity of the situation. There is a lot to be said for "change of scenery." It really
helped to get away from those things that could keep reminding us that things weren't as we would have chosen.**

The next weekend was my twelfth birthday. A
friend of mine asked me to go to the movie with
him and his brother. His mother came to get me,
and we went to see the movie. When they brought me
home, we walked in the back door. All of a sudden all
these people jumped out from the hall and the living
room and yelled "Surprise." I was so shocked and
pleased that I couldn't keep from smiling. In fact, I just
stood there for the longest time smiling a huge smile.
There were so many people there; it was a family party
with kids and their parents. We had Mexican food for
dinner. We jumped on the trampoline outside in the back
yard for a lot of the time. And then we went in to open
presents. I got a lot of neat stuff. I got a raft, a pillow table,
leggos, a picture Bible, and a lot of other neat stuff. I felt
very special and very loved that night. Our friends were
so great.
    Something else very special also happened on my
birthday. Mrs. Sinclair knew it was my birthday on July
16 and wanted to get me a Children's Bible like one her
son, Scott, had had when he was little. She said that she
went into Scott's room the week before my birthday to
look for his Bible so that she could make sure to get one

exactly like his. She looked and looked for a long time but she never could find it. So she decided that she would just go to a Christian book store and see if she could recognize one just like Scott's. She said that when she got in her car to leave she thought she heard a voice saying to her, "Go look."

She said she thought to herself, "That's crazy, I have already looked all over Scott's room."

So she started to back out of her driveway when she heard the voice again saying, "Just go look." She said that the voice was so real and yet she thought that she was going crazy, but she decided to go look one more time. When she got to Scott's room, his Bible was on his desk. She couldn't believe it. And what is really unbelievable is that when she was looking at it and turned to the page in the front where you write whose Bible it is and who gave it, it said, "To Scott Sinclair from his parents Elizabeth and John Sinclair, July 16th, 1976." Mrs. Sinclair said that she didn't remember when she gave Scott that Bible or why, but one thing that she knew was that July 16 didn't mean a thing to their family. It wasn't a birthday or anniversary or anything in their family. She decided to give that very Bible to me since it had my birthday written in it, and she felt that that was God's intention. I was pleased to receive it and felt it was very special since God must have wanted me to have it bad enough to lead Mrs. Sinclair to it.

The next weekend we had another terrific trip. Charlie and I went with my dad and a friend of his, Richard, in Richard's airplane and flew to Disney World in Florida. Richard took his little boy William. It was neat because again we got VIP treatment because Richard knows a guy who works in Disney World so we got free passes. It was a milestone in my life because I had always hated roller coasters and fast rides like that, but this trip I decided to be really brave and ride Space Mountain which is like a roller coaster, only neater. I rode it several times because I loved it so much. I was also very proud that I had finally gotten brave enough to ride one of those things. We spent a weekend there. On the way back, Richard let me fly the plane. He was not even touching the wheel and he showed me how to make the plane go up and down and turn. When we got back to Houston he let me help land it. That was really a thrill. It was pretty easy, but I was still nervous anyway.

August 1984

August was another really fun month. Mary Kessler came home from camp just in time to go on a family trip to Canada. My grandmother, Mimi, took us and my two uncles and their families. There were sixteen of us.

We first flew to Dallas and then to Seattle, where we changed planes to go to Vancouver. Vancouver was a blast. We got to feed the seagulls that came to our hotel windows. We got to go bicycling all around the bay. The bicycling was probably the most fun because there were a lot of hills to go up and down.

We got to go on a ferry ride and see a big market that had a lot of fish and food and fresh fruits and flowers. From our hotel window we could see cruisers coming into the bay. The air was so clean and fresh and felt great.

After a couple of days we boarded a train one night to ride to Jasper, Canada. The train trip was fun but it was long. We laughed a lot. When we finally got to Lake Louise, we then had to face a three-hour car trip to Jasper Lodge. When we arrived at Jasper Lodge there were many trays of food for us because it was late at night and we hadn't eaten in a while.

Jasper is on a beautiful lake and there are many things to do. One afternoon we rented kayaks and paddled around the lake. We each had our own canoe or kayak and we had races. It was really fun. We rode bikes,

took walks around the lake, and played games. We had
the bikes rented for the entire week, and Mary Kessler set
up a fun bike course for us that took us all around the
property. One neat thing was that we could eat in any restaurant in the lodge and charge it to our room.
    The lodge is a big golfing place, so we played golf a
lot. One day when we had finished a round, we went
back to the golf shop to return our clubs. We found out
that one of my clubs was missing, so my dad and I went
out to the course to find it. We came to this older couple
who had found it. After they gave us the club, the man
started saying what a fine looking boy I was and started
rubbing the top of my head. My hair started falling out
again, and it started flying everywhere, but the man
didn't seem to notice because he kept on rubbing and saying how fine I was. It was really funny, and my dad and I
had to keep from laughing out loud. We hoped that he
didn't have allergies because if he did he was going to
start sneezing and coughing and he wouldn't know why.
When we got back to the cabin where everyone was, we
told them the story, and we all had a good laugh. The
poor man probably still doesn't know what he did.
    We also took a tram car halfway up the mountain and
then hiked the rest of the way up. It was a very long hike
and very tiring but a lot of fun.
    Every night after dinner we all piled in our cars and
went looking for bears. We almost always saw them because at night they would come out and go through all the
garbage at the lodge. We chased one of them up a tree. It
was fascinating to watch them. They were big black bears
who were more afraid of us than we were of them. But the
people who live there did warn us to be on the lookout
when we were walking outside at night. It was sort of an
eerie feeling but a lot of fun.
    I did so well on the whole trip that we decided that
they must have mixed my x-rays up with poor ol' Bob
Neihouse's x-rays again; that he must be the one with the
stuff in his lungs and liver. How could anyone look and
feel as great as I did and have such a serious illness?

When we returned to Houston, I had to be in the hospital the next day for chemo. I was not looking forward to that because it was the same treatment that made me so sick before. We again had to wait all day, and finally they started the eight-hour treatment at 6:00 that night. My mom was tired and very depressed that we had to wait so long after wasting a whole day waiting for them to get started. And sure enough I got very sick for the whole night. My mom had to stay awake to help me when I got sick, so she didn't get to go to sleep at all. She cried almost all night while I slept; I woke up only to get sick and she had to help me each time that I got sick. It was an awful two days.

This was the roughest time that Bo had ever had in the hospital. It was the roughest on Larry and me as well. Bo's description of the day was very accurate. The night was equally horrible because Bo would vomit every half hour and I would have to turn his head to the side or he might choke. Therefore, neither one of us got any real uninterrupted sleep. This was the only time in all of his illness that I really became hysterical. I was there in the dark, all alone with Bo, who was so very sick, and I cried as hard as I have ever cried. And I was mad at God. I kept thinking that He supposedly never gives us more than we can handle, but I believed He had misjudged my limit this time. The only time Bo had been awake in the last twelve hours was to throw up. When he heard me and I told him what was wrong, that I was mad at the doctors and that I was mad at God, he said to me, "It is not for us to decide how long or how hard God's test is to be — it is only our responsibility to endure it." And he then went back to sleep.

If I had not been there to hear it, I would not have believed it. He said it so profoundly, with such meaning. I really had to believe that it was God speaking through him, trying to make me understand. I'm not sure I understood, but I did stop my uncontrollable sobbing. I did feel calmer than I had felt in awhile.

September 1984

And then we went to the bay for Labor Day weekend. I took a couple of my friends to the bay. I raced in the Labor Day series (sailing my sunfish). I did not do too well, and I lost my temper. So after one of the races I jumped out of my boat and I was really cussing. I was really mad.

The next day we had a family hot dog party at our bay house because we had just finished remodeling the bay house. On Labor Day we always have an awards ceremony for the end of the summer. The neatest award that a kid can get is called the "Ben Cash" award for good sportsmanship or simply for being a nice guy. I really wanted to get that award, but I didn't think that I would get it because I had lost my temper the day before in the race. All the children voted on it, not any adults. They always announce it at the very end, so I had to wait for all the other awards to be given. When they finally announced that I had won, I just sat there afraid that maybe I had heard wrong. My friends had to push me up to the front to accept it. Everyone cheered and clapped, and they took a lot of pictures of me. It made me feel so proud and loved and appreciated. I was very appreciative. They gave me a huge trophy which has all the other winners' names engraved on it. I was to have my name engraved on it and I get to keep it for a year. My dad's name was on it because he had won it when he was my age and so had my cousin Kimberly. It meant a lot to all of us.

That next week was the beginning of school. I was a little nervous the first day because I was being held back a grade since I had missed so much school the year before. I was repeating fifth grade. My friend Braden was coming over in the morning to go to class with me so that I wouldn't have to walk into class alone. It turned out that nobody acted surprised or asked questions, and I knew most of the children in the new class already. I was shy and didn't talk to many people the first couple of days, but then it got easier. When I got home the first day I was so excited about my class and told my mom all about it; I just knew that it was going to be a great year.

One special friend that was in my new class was a boy named George Biggs. He was close to God like I felt I was, and he was brave because he wasn't afraid of what to say to me because I had cancer. He also made me feel especially welcome to the fifth grade when I joined the class. He joined my scout troop, and we did a lot together. He cared about people a lot.

His family was having a concert for a man named Don Francisco, a Christian singer who is from Colorado. It was a beautiful concert of all Christian songs in Jones Hall, a large auditorium in Houston. My whole family was to attend, but George invited me to go as his special guest. I got to sit in the front row and I got to go backstage with George and meet the musicians before and after the concert and during intermission. The concert was a truly wonderful experience, and you could feel God's love for everyone throughout the auditorium. Everyone left with such a happy feeling. I then spent the night at George's house.

The next morning we went on a scout campout together. It was a special campout for me because I earned my Tenderfoot rank in scouts. I had been working on that award for about a year. I was so excited.

One bad thing happened in September that really shook me up. My grandfather, Big Daddy, went into the hospital for some tests because he had had blood in his urine. They discovered that he had a large malignant tumor in his bladder. They removed it. When my mom told me, I burst into tears because I couldn't stand to see it happen to another member of my family. My mom told me that his cancer wasn't as bad as mine and that it was a hopefully curable type. She also said, "Whatever happens, Bo, it's going to be okay, remember?"

I smiled and said, "Well it looks like Big Daddy and I are going to be in a race to see who gets to heaven first."

Later that week my mom said that the pathology report came back and that the doctor was sure that they had gotten it all and that he wouldn't even have to have chemo. I replied, "I guess there'll be a slight delay in the race." We laughed.

Big Daddy seemed to recover from his surgery pretty quickly, and I was sure glad that he didn't have to have chemo and everything that goes with it. So was he!

October 1984

On October 8, I officially received my Tenderfoot neckerchief and pin for my scout uniform at the Court of Honor ceremony. It was thrilling to me to finally have it officially because I had really worked hard to earn it. It showed me that the things that you should be most proud of are the things that you have to work for. George became an official Boy Scout that night.

One night my family went out to dinner on the way to the bay for the weekend. We started talking about Halloween and what we should be. We began making up some funny ideas and started laughing hysterically. We had all just seen the movie "Ghostbusters" so we decided to be "Pumpkin Busters." It was a really fun time, and after we got home from the bay we began working on our costumes. All six of us were dressed alike.

We had a neighborhood party and B. J. Willingham, our good friend who lives down the street, roasted a huge pig and we had all sorts of other food. We then went trick or treating as a whole group. There were a lot of people, and it was the most fun Halloween that we've ever had.

November 1984

In November I didn't have chemo because my blood counts were too low. I was glad to miss it. One Friday afternoon George was at my house to play football with my brother and his friends. After the football game we were jumping on the trampoline playing another game. All of a sudden I fell on the trampoline and I was sweating a lot and I couldn't move my legs. I had a hard time getting inside, and I told George that I couldn't play anymore. My parents weren't home at the time, and I was terrified. I prayed that my parents would show up quickly and almost instantly my mom drove up. Charlie told my mom where I was and my mom dashed into the den and found me lying on the couch. We were supposed to be leaving on a hunting trip with our friends the Stewarts. We had a hard time deciding whether or not to go on and go. We decided to go ahead and go. My leg was still hurting but not quite as badly and continued to hurt all through the weekend. But we still had a great time. Charlie and I both shot some birds. It was a fun trip.

We knew that at some point Bo's physical condition (which was excellent to this point) would begin to deteriorate. It was simply a matter of time, but we didn't know when. Nobody knew when — we just knew that it would.

When I arrived home that particular afternoon, and Charlie alerted me that Bo had a problem, something told me "This is it." I was able to calm him by my usual "you're okay." (How many times did I say those words in the past two years? And I was saying them for both of us — it seemed to make us both feel better.)

The pain seemed to diminish somewhat, after awhile, and since we had all been looking forward to this weekend trip, we decided to go as planned.

Bo's leg hurt him off and on all weekend, but he managed to do everything he wanted. It was the last weekend he was fully active. Somehow I suspected that it would be his last active weekend, but I also knew that it would be okay.

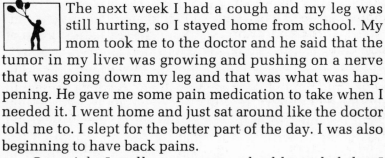 The next week I had a cough and my leg was still hurting, so I stayed home from school. My mom took me to the doctor and he said that the tumor in my liver was growing and pushing on a nerve that was going down my leg and that was what was happening. He gave me some pain medication to take when I needed it. I went home and just sat around like the doctor told me to. I slept for the better part of the day. I was also beginning to have back pains.

One night I really got upset and told my dad that I was afraid that I was really going to die and that I didn't have much time left. He said to me, "Bo, nobody knows, except God, when anyone is going to die. But if you decide that you are indeed going to die soon and that you don't have much time left then I am going to make sure that whatever time you do have left is going to be the best time you or anybody has ever had." And with that he told me to get in the car because we were going to Toys R Us (a big toy store) and get some indoor games that we could all play. I realized how fortunate I was because there were a lot of kids who might have the same problem that I have whose parents could not afford to go and purchase new games. I felt thankful, and Dad and I had a great time.

**Larry was magnificent in his reassuring Bo. He sounded
so sure of what he was saying that it gave all of us encouragement to make the best of all of our time.**

I stopped going to PE classes because of my leg
hurting; I had PE first period so I just slept late
and went to school afterwards. My classrooms
are mainly on the second floor, so I had to walk up the
stairs and it really took a lot out of me to do it. By the end
of the day I was always exhausted. By the end of the first
quarter I was only going to school for a couple of hours a
day. And when the second quarter started, I was in too
much pain to go at all. I spent most of the day at home
watching TV and working on this book.

I got the idea of writing this book at about the time I
had to stop going to school. An author of children's books
came to River Oaks Baptist to talk about how you write
books and while I was listening to her, the idea came into
my head. At first I was too embarrassed to tell anyone
what I wanted to write about, so I told my parents that I
was going to write a story that I made up. Finally, I decided to tell my parents what I really wanted to write
about and they said that they thought it would be wonderful and that it might help others.

So that night I wrote one page. I showed it to my parents and they thought it was the best that I had ever done.
I had had learning disabilities since I was in second grade
and not only that, I had the most unreadable handwriting
you've ever seen. So when my parents saw that not only
could they read what I had written, but that there was not
one mistake on the page, they said that maybe God made
it that way to tell me that I should really write this book.
And each page that I wrote after the first continued to be
pretty good, by my standards. I still hated the writing part
though because it took me so long. Eventually, I began
dictating to my parents, first on a tape recorder and then

my mom typed on her typewriter. Finally, we got a word processor and that is what we use today.

Sometimes my brother and sister had a hard time really understanding what was happening to me. We all seemed to be fighting and calling each other names and hurting each other for no reason. One night at the dinner table my mom said she wanted us all to have a talk. First she wanted all of us to go around the table and tell what really makes us angry or what really hurts our feelings. (Mary Kessler had gone up to bed because she had the flu.) Alexandra really just listened without saying anything. Charlie said that it hurt his feelings when we called him fat. And I said that it hurt my feelings when someone teased me about my bald head. So my mom said that she hoped that we all loved each other enough that we would respect each other's feelings and make sure we didn't tease each other about something that we knew hurt the other's feelings. Charlie and I agreed that we would try. Then my dad said he wanted to know what each of us was feeling about my situation, my illness, and the fact that I might die. Charlie became very quiet and finally he burst into tears with his head in my mother's lap, sobbing uncontrollably. We had been trying to make him talk about it but he never would open up. Finally he sat up, still crying, and said that he was very worried about me and what would happen to our family if I died. My mom said, "Charlie, first of all, God is the only one who knows how this is all going to turn out."

Then Charlie said, "But if he does die what will we do? What will I do? Who's going to help me with my leg-gos and play baseball with me?" It was really sad.

My mom said, "If Bo does die we know that Bo will be okay; he'll be in heaven. The rest of us will be very sad and we will cry, but we will be sad and we will cry to-gether as a family and it will be okay. And Bo will always be a part of our family. We are lucky that we have lots of pictures of all of us having many fun times together and we have so many wonderful memories and Bo will always be a part of those memories. And someday when we all die, we will all be together in heaven." And my mom kept saying, "It's going to be okay no matter what happens."

Poor Charlie still was upset and kept looking at me. So I finally told him, "What Mom said is true, Charlie, it's all going to be okay. I will be happier than I have ever been and you can be happy for me. And you are going to be okay too, even if you do cry, because everyone cries at different times and it's okay to cry. It makes you feel better if nothing else."

We all cried and then we all felt better.

Later that week Mary Kessler came into my parent's room. She seemed like she had something on her mind and finally she started crying for the same reason Charlie had cried. She said that she didn't know how our family would be without me if I died. My mom said to her, "Well one way I try to look at it is like when I ship you off to camp for the summer. I miss you so much but then I think of how very happy you always are at camp and that helps take away the hurt of missing you, just knowing how happy you are. So we must try to think of Bo as being at 'camp' and so very happy."

"But he won't be coming home to us like I always come home."

"That is true, but we will see him again when we all get to heaven and we can look forward to that." They talked some more, and I think that Mary Kessler felt better afterwards. Talking about something always seems to help rather than keeping it inside of you. If you keep it inside of you too much, you sometimes feel like you might pop.

When I heard my mom telling someone about these two conversations, she said that God had really helped her choose the right words to say.

During these two years, we had learned and were still learning how to share our feelings and emotions. Larry and I

felt that it was very important to allow our children to see our bad times as well as our good times. And it was equally important for them to share their feelings with each other. The expression "misery loves company" is very true and very applicable in this kind of situation. It is always nice to know that you aren't the only one feeling afraid or sad or lonely. Several times a week, Larry and I, at appropriate times, would ask each individual leading questions to help them expose their feelings. Sometimes it was easy, sometimes not, but from everything we had read, we felt it important to at least try.

The word "death" became part of our vocabulary. We didn't dwell on it, by any means, but we became comfortable with it and this is something that I hope we never lose. Death is the only guarantee any of us have in this life, and yet it is the one thing that we most avoid talking about. From practically the minute a child is conceived, we talk about the impending birth of the child. For nine months we prepare for it and everyone related feels comfortable about it. Birth is a passage in this life. Isn't death, then, another passage? So why do we not talk about it? It is just as important as birth, and probably more so.

I believe one of the greatest gifts we can give our children is to relieve them of the fear of death, to teach them that death is not the worst thing that can ever happen to us, and to prepare them. After all, God is the only one who knows when He will call one of his children home.

I felt very guided when we had our intimate discussions, and they left me with the warmest of feelings.

On Sunday, November 11, there was a parade held in my honor. Our friends and neighbors, the Willinghams, the D'Antonis, and the Hannahs, bought a parade to be given in my honor. It was sold at a Junior League auction by about twenty couples. The parade was about twenty cars long and all the cars were painted or decorated with all sorts of things. My favorite float was a car decorated like a shark, and it had a sign on it that said "Jaws." We were a little late getting started because a reporter from the *Houston Chronicle* was taking pictures and getting information about me. I was in the lead float, which was a very old fire engine. I got to wear a real fireman's hat, which they let me keep. There were two policemen on two motorcycles escorting the whole parade. They made traffic stop while we were coming through. We left from the Junior League building and drove down a main street to get to our neighborhood. When we arrived in our neighborhood, there were hundreds of people lining the streets waving and cheering us on. There were whistles and horns blowing and sirens screaming. It was so exciting. And these people were clapping and waving at me and the rest of my friends who were riding with me. And then the parade went to our neighborhood park where there were clowns and a "tall" man on hidden stilts. They were passing out bubble gum and balloons and things like that. There was all sorts of "junk food." The two policemen let me ride on the back of one of the motorcycles. That was a blast. And after I had ridden the motorcycle, the other policeman wrote out a ticket in my name.

It was funny. I was a little nervous around the policemen.

A few days later the reporter, Betty Ewing, called my mom to get some more information on me. They talked for a pretty long time. The next Sunday there was a full-page article on me and my parade and my book in the *Houston Chronicle*. There was a half-page full-color photograph of me in the fire truck with Charlie and my other friends who rode in the truck. It was a wonderful article, and again I felt like a hero. I couldn't believe that I had been in the paper twice in two years. That was really a thrill.

We had a wonderful Thanksgiving down at the bay. We invited our friends the Uptons (and my godmother, Ginger) for the weekend. While we were there I got worried about how much my legs hurt and how weak they were getting. I wondered how I was going to get places. My mom and dad told me that legs are a luxury that we usually just take for granted and that there was not one place on this earth that they couldn't get me to if we wanted. That made me feel a little better, I guess, but I still wished that I could be outside participating in sports and things. But as I had learned and was learning, life isn't always as easy as we would like.

Our Thanksgiving dinner was a feast just like the pilgrims had. We ate outside because it was a beautiful, perfect day. I believe that everyone there felt very, very grateful that day that we were all together. At least I know I did. The Friday after Thanksgiving we went to Galveston. (Galveston is only a twenty-minute drive from our bay house.) It turned out to not be a whole lot of fun because my leg was hurting too much for me to keep up with everyone. We didn't stay in Galveston for very long.

The rest of the weekend was a lot of fun. I just sat around but so did everyone else, and it was fun just being with my family and friends.

December 1984

In December I stayed at home a lot and worked on my book. This was when we got a home computer and my mom's friend, deSha, taught her how to put the book into the word processor. It made it a lot more fun for my mom because she could correct her mistakes as soon as she made them.

My cousin Laura came home from Germany for the Christmas holidays. She was home early in December before anyone else had gotten out of school, so she came over during the school day to visit. It was nice having company early in the day when everyone else had to be in school.

I also made Christmas presents out of clay for people in my family. (My mom and Aunt Eckie have kilns so we could fire our things.) My mom decided that she was going to make all of her presents for everyone because she didn't feel like going to a bunch of stores. We all have too much anyway, and we wanted to focus on the real meaning of Christmas — giving and not receiving in Jesus Christ's name. It made it a lot of fun because everyone in my family except my dad was making things out of clay.

I was not having chemo anymore because it wasn't doing any good and I felt too awful to have it. We were turning it all over to God and felt that He would do whatever he saw best for us. I hoped we were doing the right thing; I felt like we were. My mom had to keep reminding me that God could see much farther than we could, and we just had to trust him.

And it sure made me appreciate the time that I had on this earth. I did get afraid of dying a lot more than I used to. I guess it was becoming more real to me and my family; I really and truly might die from this! But then we would talk about it and realize that if I did die it would be okay; I would be the lucky one in heaven with God and Jesus and it would be a perfect life for me.

I just hoped that it wouldn't hurt too much. My mom always told me that there was nothing to be afraid of for us Christians about dying. The only fear was the pain, and medicine could take care of that. And the rest would be wonderful — to live in a perfect place where there was no pain, no lines to wait in, no guilt or jealousy, no threats of nuclear war, and no cancer or other awful diseases. This made me feel a lot better, almost excited. It was like going on a fabulous trip.

Every time we went to the doctor we would get more bad news. The tumor in my liver was growing larger and larger and you could now see it. The doctor told me that my leg would probably not get any better. That really upset me. But I thought to myself, "I can't let it ruin my life, whatever life I had left. I had to make the best of my time that I could and that it would not do me a bit of good to sit around feeling sorry for myself." So I learned to enjoy watching people participate in sports and watching other activities. It wasn't so bad once I got used to it.

Back in September I decided that I would ask for a new bike for Christmas. But as it neared Christmas, I realized that I would probably never ride a bike again because of my leg and it would be stupid to ask for a bike. So I asked for and received a piano keyboard and a lot of leggo blocks. I built a whole town of leggos.

Christmas Day was probably the most wonderful Christmas we have ever had. Usually my mom and dad have to figure out whose family we will have Christmas dinner with — my mom's or my dad's. So one night before Christmas, in the middle of the night, I went into my parents' room because my leg was hurting. My mom and dad and I sat up and talked in my parents' bed. My mom said they had decided that we weren't going to go to anyone's house for dinner, that for the first time in my life we were going to stay at our own house. (The reason was that I was feeling weaker and weaker and they didn't think that I could sit up long enough to sit through a formal meal at someone else's house.) And my dad agreed and said that if anyone wanted to see us, they could come see us at our house. So I said, "You mean there's not going to be any 'Come on Bo, quit unwrapping your presents, you can finish when we get home,' or 'Come on Mumu (Mary Kessler), you can call Sharon back later,' or 'Hurry up Charlie, you have to take a bath,' or 'No Ali (Alexandra) you can't take all your Barbie dolls to Mimi's'?" That was how every Christmas morning was at our house. We were always in a hurry to get to someone's house for Christmas dinner. I was excited at the idea of being at home all day long. And it turned out to be a fabulous day.

After we opened our presents and played for a while we had lunch. My mom had prepared a huge lunch of turkey and dressing and everything that goes with it. We each said a blessing at the table (and the blessings were beautiful) and gave God thanks for everything He had given us over the past years. Then Alexandra went to the kitchen and got some bread and started passing it and some wine. She said the blessing that the priests always do at church when they are giving communion: "The body of Christ, the bread of heaven." She said it perfectly. It was real cute, but we all took it seriously also. We were all feeling close to God. It was a very special lunch. It showed us that it was much more meaningful to live the real meaning of Christmas instead of worrying about what you get or don't get.

The whole day was one to behold. We really could feel God's presence, especially during lunch. I remember sitting at the table, looking at my husband and children and feeling ecstatic. And then I thought to myself: "Here I have a dying child who can barely sit up at the table — God only knows what traumas are ahead for us — and, yet, I feel nothing but joy." It didn't make a bit of sense, and then I realized it's that old phrase that I mentioned earlier — "the peace that passeth all understanding." It's not meant to be understood or to make sense. It's a gift that only God can give, and it's always there; we just have to ask for it and accept it.

 My sister, Mary Kessler, spent most of Christmas vacation with me. She had been invited to go to Mexico with a friend but didn't go because she was worried that something might happen to me and she wanted to be home in case it did. She played games with me, indoor games that I could play. She was always very careful to see if I were comfortable enough or if I needed anything. We just spent a lot of time visiting and talking, something that we had not done in a long time. She and I had always been close, and it made me feel good that that had not changed.

We went back to the bay for New Year's weekend. The Uptons came and our friends, the Geises, from Colorado. We had gone out to buy some fireworks. When we got back into the car all of a sudden I got real dizzy and felt like I was going to throw up. My legs, both of them, started hurting so badly, and then I lost feeling in my legs and in my feet. My toenails started turning blue. It was very scary. My mom called the doctor back in town, and he said that he thought the tumor was affecting more nerves in my leg and to try to keep my legs elevated. He also said that I could take more pain medication than I had been taking. Somehow we still managed to have a fun time.

Bo and I talked a lot about death at this point. He seemed to have a lot more questions and seemed to need reassurance about what it would be like. He didn't appear afraid; it was more of a curiosity. It was very easy to talk about it with him, and he seemed to grasp every word that I said. I have to say that it made me a lot more comfortable with the subject also, as I was beginning to realize quite plainly that death really is simply a part of life and it really isn't anything to fear. One day when we had been working on the book, he decided that he wanted to do something a little different. He wanted to tell me what he thought heaven would be like. The following is what he wrote:

"LIFE AND DEATH"

We were put on this earth because God had so much love that he wanted to share it with everyone. He put us on this earth for a purpose; each person has a different purpose and each person has a different talent or gift that God has given him to use for this purpose. I think I found my purpose. My purpose is to spread Jesus' love to everybody. My gift is my sense of humor (so my parents have told me) and I am to use this gift to make other people happy and to laugh.

Things I like about this world: I like sunny days that only have a few clouds in the sky; I like laughing a lot; I loved participating in sports and since I can't participate in them anymore, I love watching them; I like feeling good; I like going on trips with my family; I like talking to God, it helps you to know Him better and it gives you a good feeling inside — in fact, I have talked to God so much that I now forget to bow my head because I am so used to just simply talking to Him.

I look forward to getting out of this (cancer) one way or another. I can't decide which way I want out of it — either way I win. I am looking forward to the next world if I don't make it in this world.

When you die it is like a dream with bright lights all over the place. It is like being in a bright and beautiful forest. And I picture Jesus' face — a peaceful face which is looking for you to follow His word. He is real glad to see you. When you get to heaven everyone is so happy there and are clapping and cheering and so glad to have you be there with them. You have a perfect feeling. It's like when you get out of a bathtub and you are all clean and comfortable — well, you feel even better than that.

This is what I want to happen to my body when I die: I want to be cremated because the heat out of the furnace will rise and your spirit will get to heaven that much faster. And it will also make sure you are dead. One reason that I do not like funerals is because everyone stands around and cries and is sad. If I should die any time soon, I want balloons, a lot of helium balloons, and firecrackers, because I want it to be a real celebration. God would want it that way and therefore so do I. And I don't want anyone to cry, but to be happy for me.

January 1985

In early January Big Daddy had to go back into the hospital for more surgery. This time they found nine tumors in his bladder. We were all sorry that they had found more cancer because this meant that they would have to do some form of chemotherapy on him. But the doctor told him that this kind of chemotherapy was going to be very mild and would have no side effects; he wouldn't get sick or lose his hair. He had to have it once a week for six weeks. I was sure sorry for him to have to go through it. But he seemed to do just fine.

January was about the same as the last couple of months, but not as busy. My mom and I had a lot more time to work on my book. I went to visit my PE class one time, and it was fun seeing my friends. My friend, George Biggs, still came to visit me a lot. He was a very loyal friend to me. He would come to visit me in the afternoons and sometimes I didn't feel like seeing him but that didn't discourage George. He would just sit with me; sometimes we'd talk and he'd tell me what was going on at school. Other times he would just sit with me and not say anything. It made me feel good just knowing he was there. A good friend is a gift from God and is worth everything.

My other friends from school constantly sent me letters and cards and sometimes, several times a week, someone would show up with cookies.

My mom's birthday was January 16. We celebrated her birthday at home at dinnertime when my dad got home from work. Charlie presented my mom a cake that he and Ganga (my grandmother) had gotten that afternoon at the grocery store. My mom thought it was one from her favorite bakery and said how excited she was. It really hurt Charlie's feelings because he hadn't gotten it at the bakery. When my mom realized what she had done, she made a big deal about his giving her the cake and how thrilled she was to have any cake, so we all ate it. Charlie was having a bad time emotionally at that time and was extra sensitive. He was mainly worried about me. I kept trying to tell him that everything was going to be okay no matter what happened to me, but he was still worried.

About that time we started seeing a psychiatrist named Betty. The first time I saw her I felt very uncomfortable, but each time it got easier and I always felt better after I had visited with her. The first time I went to her, she asked me a lot of questions. She asked if I were afraid of dying, and I said that I wasn't because I knew it would be perfect. She asked what I meant by perfect, and I told her like a wonderful dream that you don't ever want to wake up from. She asked me how I knew that, and I told her that the Bible told us that and I believe everything that the Bible told me. I also told her how close to God I had gotten over the past two years and how I knew he would heal me either in this life or the next. I also told her that it was true that everyone who believed in Christ as our Savior would be given the gift of eternal life just as I would. She seemed very interested.

On the way home my mom told me that it was beautiful the way I said what I said. I then asked my mom if Betty were a Christian. My mom said that she didn't think so because her last name was Levine and that is a Jewish name. I asked mom why I was seeing a non-Christian psychiatrist and my mom said, "Maybe God has led you to her so that you can teach her about Christ."

I said, "If that is the case, when is she going to start paying me instead of my paying her?" We laughed.

I began going to see her twice a week; once by myself and once with my brother and sisters. I really enjoyed going because after visiting with her I always seemed to feel a little better. And she helped our family to get along better.

In this type of situation, there are times that it is harder to care for the other children than to care for the patient. The patient has everyone's attention and has total control over everyone, whereas the other family members feel neglected, even resentful. Hardly a day went by that someone didn't bring something for Bo. The other three children were beginning to feel the strain that we had been feeling plus every time the doorbell rang, they knew that it was something else for Bo. We finally had to ask that people not bring things just to Bo; things that the children could share were fine. We just couldn't risk their ultimately resenting Bo. This most likely irritated some people, but we had to take that chance and do what we thought best for our immediate family. After all, we were the ones who were living with this situation, day in and day out, and could see the possible repercussions. We realized that those who had never been in this situation could not begin to understand what we were going through, but we hoped that they could at least respect our feelings. The doctors told us early in the illness that we had to think of our family first and always do what we thought beneficial to everyone as a whole.

 My family has always loved to laugh, and if we all hadn't kept our senses of humor over the past two years, I don't think we could have made it. Laughter is another gift from God, and we had been blessed with a lot of laughter.

One day my dad and I were going to go to school to my PE class so I could see my friends. I didn't tell my dad until we got to school that my shoulder was hurting a lot. I felt pretty bad, but I was anxious to see everyone. I wasn't very friendly because I felt so crummy, but the kids didn't seem to mind. It was good to see them. When I got home I told my mom that I couldn't believe how loving those kids were to me and it made me feel so great.

A few days later, Mr. O'Keefe came over to my house and brought me another huge trophy. (Remember that he had brought me a Christian trophy back in May of 1983.) He told me that when I first became sick, he believed that life was the most important thing in the world but that I had taught him that there was something more important on this earth and that was our accepting God's plan. This trophy had my name on it and also engraved on it was a verse from Romans. It was Romans 8:37, which says, "We are more than conquerors through Him who loved us." It had three crosses on it, two small ones on each side and one large one in the middle. Mr. O'Keefe stayed a long time and visited with us, and I was glad to see him.

The next weekend I went to see my friends again at a birthday party. It was a bowling party. I was sitting in my wheelchair watching everyone bowl when a man that I didn't know came up to me and asked me why I wasn't bowling. I didn't really know what to say to him, but I just said my legs hurt if I stand up. He told me that that was no excuse, that there were other ways to bowl, and he set up a ramp for me. I then bowled from my wheelchair. It was a ramp for the handicapped; the handicapped people use it every Saturday. I did really well from my chair and was very pleased.

One day my mom was at Eckie's house when she noticed on her bulletin board there was a tiny little scratch sheet of paper with the name "Ford Atkinson" written on it. My mom knew the name because he is a reporter for television and had called my mom about two years before about doing a story on me. (He had heard about me from a friend.) For some reason they never got together about it and it was forgotten. When my mom asked Eckie why she had his name on her bulletin board, Eckie told her that our Aunt Laura whom Eckie had visited in London had mentioned him to her. Aunt Laura told Eckie that he is a distant cousin of ours and that he lived in Houston and that we should look him up. I couldn't believe it. When I told Eckie the story of his calling me two years earlier, she couldn't believe it either. She then picked up the phone and called him and invited him for dinner, explaining who she was. It turned out that he is my grandfather's cousin once removed and he is a Christian as well, and we all figured that his doing a story on me was meant to be. Anyway, we met him and enjoyed getting to know him. And then we didn't hear from him for a few weeks so my mom decided that maybe he wasn't interested in doing the story. But then he called and came over to visit. We then set up a time.

February 1985

Ford came over one afternoon with a photographer named Paul. It was amazing to see all the work that goes into filming a news story. Paul spent a lot of time putting up lights and arranging and rearranging things just so. We did all the filming in my mom's and dad's bedroom because that is where the computer is and the story that Ford was doing was about my book and how my mom and I were writing it. Paul filmed my mom typing on the computer while I talked. We did the same segment over three times. The first time he filmed me telling the story about the little boy in church telling his mother that I was baldheaded. Then he filmed my mom typing the story as I told it. The third time he filmed the monitor on the computer as my mom typed. My mom was very nervous typing while somebody was taking pictures and she made lots of mistakes. But we knew that they would not use even one half of the film that they were shooting.

Then Ford sat down and started asking me some questions. He asked me if I was afraid to die. I told him no, that I knew I would be in a better life with God and Jesus and it would be paradise. I also said that I just hoped that my family would be okay afterwards and not worry.

He then asked, "Bo, have you in the last year ever gotten mad and angry that this has happened to you?"

I said, "No, I figured that someone had to do it and I am just sorta proud that God chose me."

He asked me what I hoped to accomplish with my book — what did I want people to get out of it?

I answered, "I hope it helps people get closer to God and to learn to trust in God. And I hope that it might bring someone to Christ who doesn't know Him."

My mom said afterwards that she couldn't believe the things that I said and that I didn't seem nervous. I told her that I prayed about it before the interview and this was what God led me to say.

Ford asked me a lot more questions but then I got tired. I was also beginning to hurt, so my mom gave me some pain medication. And then Ford interviewed my mom.

He asked her what she had learned from this experience and she answered that I was a lot tougher than she would imagine she would be in the same situation. She also said that she obviously hoped that I would survive but that if I didn't that she knew God would help them get through it and that I would always be a part of this family. And that she was very proud of me.

The whole filming part took about three hours, and by the end we were all exhausted but very glad we had done it. Ford said that it would probably be on the 10:00 news that weekend. We alerted everyone to watch and then, much to our disappointment, it was not on. They did show it the next week but they didn't give us a lot of warning, so we couldn't tell everyone. But my mom and dad and grandparents were here and watched it. My two grandmothers cried and said they loved it and that they were very proud of me. I was embarrassed to admit it, but I was proud too. And a lot of other people saw it and we received many phone calls and letters from people we knew and some we didn't know. The letters we received from people we didn't know made us feel that we had touched some lives that we hadn't expected to touch. One letter that was interesting was from a man who had lived in China and spoke Chinese. He wrote that he was glad to have finally gotten to meet me even if it was on TV because he had been praying for me for the past two years. He then went on to tell me that "Bo" in Chinese means "widely read." We hoped that meant that my book would be widely read. Another letter was from a mother of another cancer patient who had just returned home with her son after spending a day at the hospital while he had radiation treatments. She said that they had just turned on the TV in time to see me, and it gave her son a lot of encouragement in believing in God. That is what I had hoped to accomplish. It made me so happy.

Bo really opened up to Ford. Eckie and I watched him being interviewed, and we were amazed at how easily he spoke and how convincing he was. Ford was terrific in handling Bo and the subject matter, and the whole segment came across as a real tribute to God. Larry and I felt a real pride in our son.

It was Valentine's Day. A couple of things happened that made it a fun day. One thing that happened was that I had a surprise visitor, Earl Campbell. The way that it happened was that there was a man named Mr. Pizzatola that I had met one day when I was having chemo in the clinic. He was there with his son who was the same age as I. His son had had leukemia and had done very well and was now off chemo; he was at the clinic for a checkup only. The man came over to my stretcher where I was having my treatment and said that he felt led to come and pray with me and for me. My mom said that it was okay, but at the time I was so sick I didn't really care what he did. The morning of February 14, Mr. Pizzatola called and said that he wanted to come by and see me. My mom said fine. When he came, he brought Earl Campbell, who used to play with the Houston Oilers. And with Earl was his little boy, Christian. I was excited because I had never met him but I had watched him on TV a lot. My mom took pictures of me with Earl and also Riri, our housekeeper, with Earl. I don't know who was more excited, me or Riri. I really wanted to go to my class party, so my mom drove me up to the school. When I got there and saw all the steps, I realized that I couldn't go up the steps; I just couldn't make it. So my mom went to my classroom and gave the kids my valentines for me. A few minutes later my mom returned to the car along with some of my classmates. They brought me some cookies and punch from the party. They also brought me a sack full of valentines and a huge poster that said, "We love you Bo," and they had all signed it. It was a very special day for me and once again I felt very loved and very happy. They really made me feel like a hero. And when I arrived home someone had sent some big red balloons and someone else had brought some brownies. It made for a very fun day.

March 1985

Bo began a sharp decline the last week of February. He could hardly sit up because his abdomen was so enlarged plus he had acute edema in his lower limbs. But incredibly enough, his spirit remained intact. He and I would go through a little ritual several times a day where I would ask him, "Bo, how are you?" to which he would reply, "My body is awful, but my spirit is great."

We discussed many times how unimportant our bodies really are and what really counts is our spirit.

 One morning I sent some donuts to my class and wrote them a letter to tell them thank you for everything they had done. This is the letter I wrote:

Dear Classmates,

Thanks for everything you've given to me and my family. The cookies and brownies have been great, and so have the cards and letters. Your thoughtfulness has made a wonderful difference in my days, they really have. I am sending you something in return and I hope you enjoy it.

Although physically I am not doing too well, my spirit and faith are great. I know that God is doing good things even though it is hard to understand sometimes.

I have learned that the body is not what's important —
what is important is your spirit and faith in God, and if
you can keep your spirit and faith way up, you know
that everything is going to be okay.
I hope that I can come visit again soon, but if I
can't, I want you to know how much your caring has
meant. Thank you.

Love,
Bo

It is now the middle of March. I can't do a lot anymore because I am weak and "physically challenged," as
I have heard young Teddy Kennedy refer to his handicap.
But now I can sit back and relax and my days aren't as
busy; I am catching a lot of life that I have missed before
and that I would have missed again had God not shown
me how to live whatever life I have left. The last few days
have been beautiful. I have spent them sitting outside
watching birds fly around and squirrels build their nests
in the trees. I have even been watching a dove's nest with
the mother and father building and caring for their young.
I think God arranged for the dove's nest to be there to
show me a sign of peace to tell me what's ahead for me. I
don't know what is ahead for me, but I have a feeling that
it is going to be great, whatever God has planned for me —
whether it's on this earth or in the next life.

The first sentence of this book refers to "another dull
day" in my life. No longer are my days "dull." I am
touched by each day because I now know how special
each day is. Thank you God.

The End

The first two weeks of March brought exceptionally mild
weather, definitely the beginning of spring. Though he could
not move his legs, Bo seemed to need less pain medication and
seemed more alert. He sat outside on a small balcony off of the
master bedroom from morning until late afternoon for several

days. Bo seemed very content and each time I, or anyone else, would come out to sit with him, he pointed out different things in the yard or the trees that he had been observing. I asked him one afternoon how he felt about his life as it was now. I asked him if he just hated sitting there all day long and if he were miserable. He looked at me with wonder that I would ask such a thing and replied, "My life is very pleasant."

I thought to myself, "His life is 'pleasant.' So are all of our lives pleasant; so why do we strive for more than pleasant? Why do we go out and buy unnecessary things and look for ways to improve our lives; why don't we settle for 'pleasant'? Bo is taking time to sit and observe things that none of us would ever take the time to do. We are much too busy, out trying to make our lives even better, than to sit and enjoy the basics of life."

Bo finished his part of the book on March 15 and was ecstatic. He really wanted to complete it, and it was as if he knew that his time was drawing near. The day that he finished it was his last good day.

Bo's last two weeks were not easy. He was in a lot more pain and never could get very comfortable. He needed his body turned from side to side every half hour, around the clock. It was spring break, and the majority of our friends had gone on their planned trips. Our sixteen-year-old niece, Palmer, with whom Bo had a very special friendship, opted to miss her family's ski trip in order to spend time with Bo. She spent many hours at our house visiting with Bo during his illness and, at the end, was there helping to physically care for him. Palmer was the one person that Bo was always happy to see, no matter how he felt, and she could always seem to make him feel better. She and our housekeeper, Riri, were an invaluable extra pair of hands those last weeks.

Bo's only other constant company was his lazy old dachshund, Raisin, who much to Raisin's delight, became a house dog for Bo's last two weeks. When Bo was in one of his few alert stages during those last weeks, he told me that he wanted a black lab puppy. (He said it with a half grin on his face.) I told him, "Bo, you know that I would do just about anything for you at this point, but here's where I have to draw the line. The last thing we need is a new puppy, and besides, you already have a dog."

Bo, with as much energy as he could muster, replied,

"Okay, Mom, let me get this straight. Here I am, a little boy who can't do anything except lie here, and I am probably going to die soon, and my own mother won't even get me a little lab puppy." I looked down to see probably the last mischievous smile from him that I would ever see again. I remember thinking to myself, "He really isn't afraid, and he's going to have a little fun down to the last minute."

My response to him was that we would make Raisin a house dog and she could stay in his bed. Raisin adjusted to her new way of life like a champ. She would lie in Bo's bed with him all day and night, leaving his side only for meals and to take short breaks outside. She thought she had indeed died and gone to heaven. And Bo loved the company.

The days and nights became a blur to Larry and me because we were up so much with Bo. But Bo never lost his spirit and never lost his faith. He must have known that his time on this earth was almost over that weekend. On Saturday night, Larry took the night shift while I slept, and while Larry was turning him, Bo told him he was sorry that he was having to take care of him. On Monday, the day he died, he told Riri how sorry he was that she was having to go through this with him. He must have known. I look forward to the day when I can ask him.

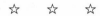

On Monday, April 1, at precisely 4:00 P.M., Bo made a magnificent and gentle landing into his next life. After many weeks of my agonizing about what the inevitable ending would be like, and when, God again revealed himself in the most glorious way. (Coincidence or not, this was also the first day of Holy week or Easter week.)

Since maintaining a relatively stable plateau since the first of March, Bo began another decline around March 28. He seemed to be in a lot more pain, he was suffering from acute edema in his limbs, and it was beginning to spread to his face. He could no longer move his legs, and he had to be turned in bed about every half hour. But his attitude was still very positive. We would still play a game where I would ask him, "Bo, how are you?" He would answer, "Physically not so great, but spiritually I am terrific." The day he died we went through that little routine. It gave me great reassurance.

On that last Monday morning, I made an appointment for 3:00 that afternoon at the clinic to see Dr. Mahoney, the doctor we had been more or less assigned to for the past few months. (Larry and I used to laugh to ourselves that this was the one and only advantage of being in the "home stretch" of this illness; you weren't shuffled among four or five doctors each time you visited the clinic. You pretty much got to see one doctor.) Anyway, Larry and I both felt that since Bo hadn't been seen in a month and seemed to be in another decline, it would be good to let the doctor have a look and give us a reading as to what was occurring.

We loaded his weak little body into the back of our Suburban and left for the hospital. Bo was miserable and begging us to take him home. If Larry or I had given in, the other would have agreed and we would have returned home. Thank God neither of us changed our minds. When we got to the hospital, we parked in the driveway between the clinic and the hospital. Bo said that he was too weak to sit up in his wheelchair, so we decided to wait in the car and intercept Dr. Mahoney when he came from the hospital on his way to the clinic. While we were waiting, Bo was mumbling something, his voice barely audible. I asked him, "What do you need, Bo? What are you saying?"

He very belligerently answered me, "I'm talking to Jesus!" It was as though he was telling us that he didn't need his earthly parents anymore, that he had found something even better.

Then Dr. Mahoney arrived and examined him. He found that Bo's pulse was considerably weaker and that his heart had slowed down. Dr. Mahoney then went with Larry to the clinic to write a prescription for morphine. He then came back by the car and stopped to tell me that Larry had gone to the pharmacy in the hospital to fill the prescription. He stayed and talked to me about Bo. He said he didn't think this could go on much longer, and we talked about our other kids and how they were doing with all this. Actually, I'm not sure about what else we talked about; I was just glad that he was staying around, hopefully until Larry got back.

The hospital pharmacy is notorious for making patients wait for long periods of time, sometimes as much as an hour for medicines, especially narcotics. Larry told the pharmacist that he would return for the drugs later because he had a sick child in the car that he needed to take home. The pharmacist replied that it would only take about five more minutes, but for some unknown reason, Larry restated that he would return later. He then came back to the car.

Two minutes later Bo took his last breath and quietly closed his eyes. Dr. Mahoney very gently listened to his heart and then said to us, "I believe the good Lord has taken him." He then warned us that Bo might start to seemingly gasp for breath or have some spasms, but he never did. There was a complete peace about him that never left after he took that last breath. Larry and I felt a surge of joy, of relief for him, and some of that same peace that our precious son had found.

The hurting and the grieving was to come — we knew that — but how could we consider this beautiful transition anything but a complete and perfect miracle? We had to be thankful for that.

I had been told many times by many people that God's timing would be perfect. I just couldn't believe how perfect it could be.

First of all, Monday, April 1, was the day after spring break was over and the majority of our close friends had just returned from trips. Two of our own children had returned on Sunday from trips with other families. My sister, Eckie, was returning from Germany that afternoon. Larry's and my being together meant a lot to both of us for obvious reasons. But it was so perfect that Larry heard Bo say that he was talking to Jesus. If I had been the only one to report it, Larry might have thought it was an exaggeration or maybe my imagination or my emotions taking over.

It gave Larry and me such security as Christian parents knowing that Bo went from our adoring arms into those of our Savior, Jesus Christ. There was no fear, no worry, no agony for him. What more could a parent ask?

God was good to Bo. And Bo never lost faith or questioned God's plan. In Bo's television interview, he was asked, "Are you mad; have you ever wondered why you've had to suffer through all this? Why not somebody else?" Bo had answered, "Well, I figured somebody had to do it, and I am sorta proud that God chose me." And this pride never left him.

Bo's memorial service was two days later, and it was very definitely the celebration he wanted. Eleven hundred people attended. We sang the most joyous Easter hymns, and our priest read the last chapter that Bo had written. (This alone would have thrilled Bo.) Had it not been against city ordinance, there would have been the requested fireworks. But there were balloons, 300 of them, at the church and at our home, that some of our loving friends sent. The day couldn't have been more perfect. I hope Bo was watching because he would have been very proud of the number of lives that he touched and of those who cared.

We have received many notes and letters from people since Bo's death, some we know and some we don't know. One person wrote, "You were blessed to have had such a unique son whom God must have sent to witness to all of us." We do feel blessed, and he was definitely a wonderful gift from God for which we will be forever thankful.

Epilogue

June 1986

It has now been over a year since Bo went to his next life. In some respects it seems like it was only yesterday and in others, it seems like it was years ago. We've obviously done a lot of reflecting on Bo's life with us. We've spent many hours thinking about his life before he became ill, during his illness, and what life is now like without him.

Bo died in April — two months before school was out for the others — which was probably a good distraction for us all. Bo's school named their field day in May in his honor. There would not be a greater honor for Bo, as this was his favorite day of the year. Larry and I attended this special event and were very moved by the 2,000 balloons sent up at the beginning of the day and 2,000 more at the closing. We felt a real sense of pride at such an honor. Yet it hurt to see all the twelve- and thirteen-year-old boys looking so vibrant and healthy. That was something I knew I would have to work through, and maybe, in time, it wouldn't be as painful.

The summer was a quiet time. I think that we were still in our shock period for most of the summer because it seemed to go so fast.

We were still in the process of learning how to cope. Bo's thirteenth birthday would have been on July 16. For the two weeks before that date, Larry and I were very depressed and finally figured that it was in anticipation of Bo's birthday. When the day finally arrived, it wasn't as painful as we had expected because we had already done most of our agonizing.

It wasn't until school began in the fall that reality hit; we were back in a structured situation, and there was definitely something missing: Bo. I read once that one of the hardest things about losing a child is that you can no longer fantasize about that child. We parents spend a good deal of time projecting into the future about what our children will do, how they will look, and so on. I never realized how much time is spent on this until that time was taken away. And when I took Charlie and Ali back to school that first day and saw Bo's class and how they had changed, I wished that I could see what Bo would look like. This was going to be one of the hardest adjustments to make.

During Bo's illness, many people seemed to feel unsure as to what to say. Larry and I could certainly sympathize with this problem, as we have been in the same position on many occasions. This problem continued after Bo's death. It's as though people were afraid to mention his name for it might remind us of him again. What people do not realize is that Bo still is on our minds all of the time. He is still such a part of our family. We have a lot of happy memories, and it brings us great joy to dwell on those memories, either alone or with others. One thing parents do not want is for any of their children to ever be forgotten, especially the one who is no longer living.

At church one Sunday, a well-meaning friend, whom I don't see too often, was asking me about Todd, my nephew, who had gone off to boarding school. She obviously had Bo on her mind as she asked me, "How's Bo doing at school?" And then, to her horror, she realized her mistake, and began apologizing profusely. I told her that it meant a lot to me that she had Bo on her mind and that he was obviously still a part of her life. She was still mortified. To mention someone's name who is no longer living is a seemingly irreversible mistake. This is a ridiculous notion. I am always thrilled when someone brings up Bo's name, even if it is only in a passing comment. It assures me that he has not been forgotten. And in visiting with other bereaved parents, I have learned that the vast majority feel the same way.

Each holiday that we faced, such as Thanksgiving and Christmas, were the same as the anticipation of Bo's birthday. We did most of the agonizing before the actual day; when the day finally arrived, it wasn't as terrible as we had expected.

We still had waves of sadness, but the waves came less frequently, and each was less intense than the one before. I believe that when one of these waves would come, it was important to ride it out, as opposed to trying to avoid it or trying to mask it. If it meant staying home all day one day every so often and crying until it hurt, that's what I did, and I encouraged the others in my family to do the same. I always seemed to feel better afterwards and was ready to proceed with my life. I think it was very important to face and to work through these emotions as long as they didn't become the dominant emotions in one's life. And now I am becoming increasingly aware that my thoughts of Bo and his life are for the most part happy thoughts, and I feel continually grateful for the twelve years we had.

In retrospect, there are probably three key items that allowed us to endure our ordeal with relative sanity and no bitterness. They are faith, humor, and openness.

Our faith that God's plan is perfect gave us a real reason to enjoy each day as it came. One has to trust that God really does know what He is doing — that He is in control. And it is a lot easier to simply trust than to try to figure out God's plan, because one can't find a solution. Our minds are too finite. Larry and I agree that when we tried to control the situation without the help of prayer, we became frustrated, angry, fearful, and tired. On the other hand, when we turned things over to God, we felt a tremendous relief — refreshed and ready to begin another day.

Humor was vital to our sanity. As important as it is to laugh during one's good times, it is even more important to be able to laugh during the bad times. We learned to laugh about irate nurses, mispronounced names, the noise of "snoring" i.v. machines, the expensive boxes of Kleenex from the hospital pharmacy, and anything else we could find to humor us. Humor kept us from expending all of our energies worrying about what tomorrow would bring.

Openness is the third essential factor. We found that people care very much and want to share the experience, but they cannot if they are not told the real status of the disease. By keeping everyone abreast of the current situation, they were much better able to understand our emotional ups and downs and thus respond to our needs. Not sharing the true situation with friends only confuses and frustrates everyone.

We learned that since people basically do care, together, with God's help, we can turn a bad situation into a loving and caring experience from which we can grow. We are all in this world together, and we have the responsibility to help each other spiritually, emotionally, and physically as long as we are on this earth.

If our most important task is to help each other to know and love God, then Bo's life had great purpose and meaning.

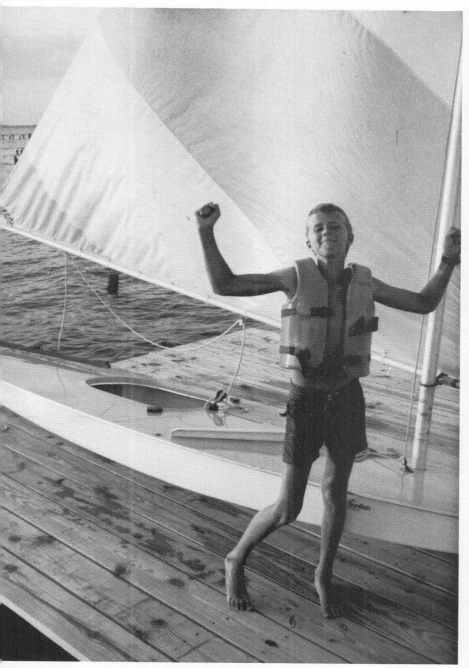

Bo after a triumphant day of sailing, on the afternoon the family found out there was no hope for his recovery, June 1984.

The Surgery

In the middle of that night I woke up scared. So we prayed about it. Then I felt better about it. The next morning I was woken up by the nurses. Before I was hardly awake. They gave me another shot in the seat. I cried, my mom cried and even my dad cried. I knew this was a dangeres oparation, because I had never seen my dad cry before. I said, "I am scared", I said. My mom said, "God will take care of you." Back then I did not trust God verry much, so I was still a little bit scared. The nurse came in to take me and we were still scared. We all laughed and then they put strecher. As I went out of my room, people I knew were lined up against the wall. I waved to all of them, but they jus

Reproduction of manuscript page in Bo's notebook.

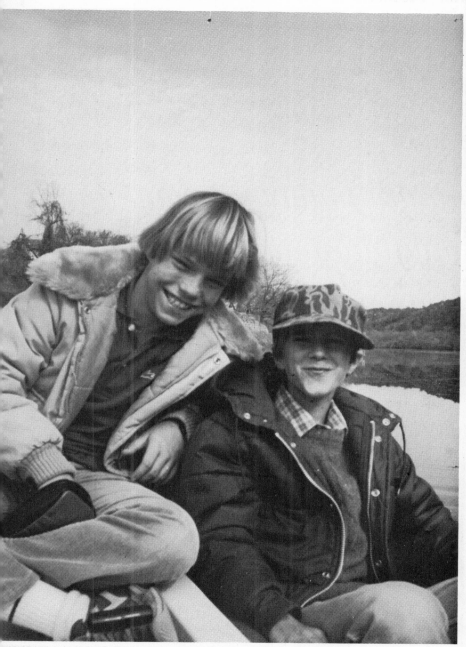

Bo with his cousin Todd Wallace (left) after one month of chemotherapy, January 1983.

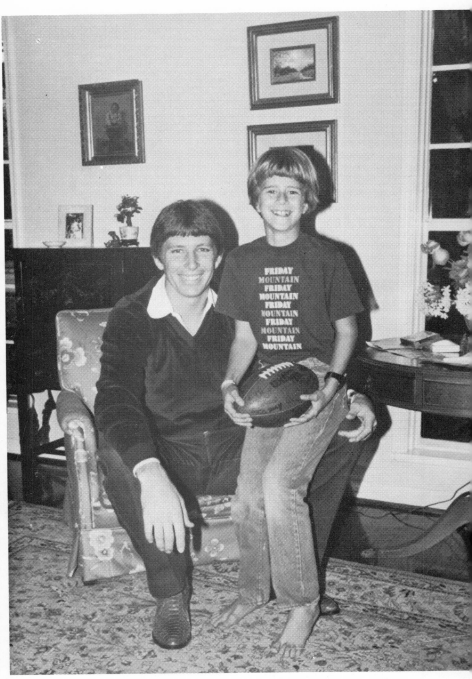

The weekend before Bo's first surgery, Houston Oilers quarterback Gifford Nielsen surprised Bo with a visit.

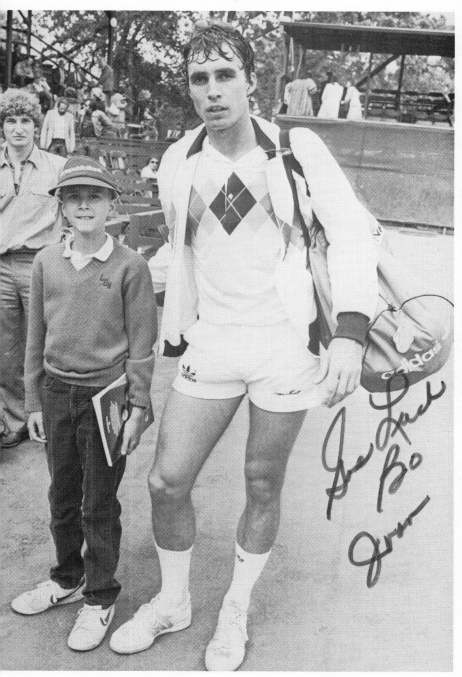

Bo meets tennis professional Ivan Lendl at a Houston
tournament.

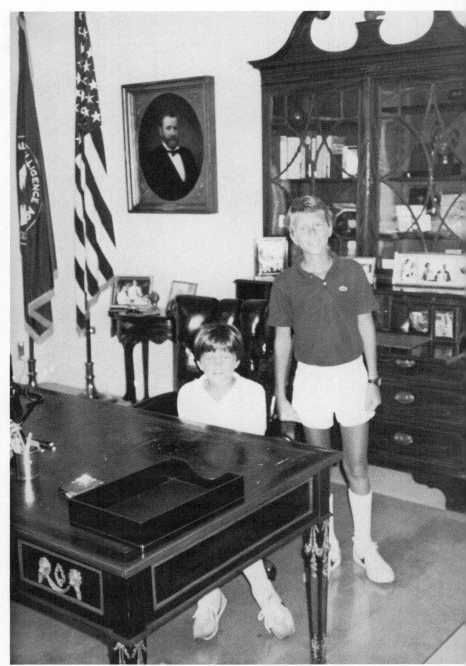

Charlie and Bo in Vice-President George Bush's office.

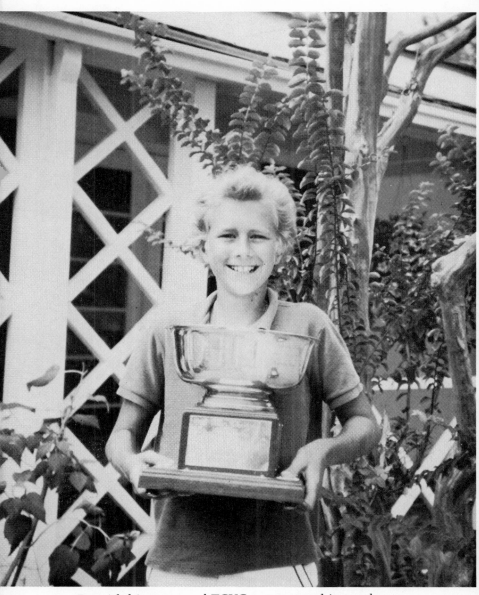

*Bo with his treasured TCYC sportsmanship trophy,
Labor Day 1984.*

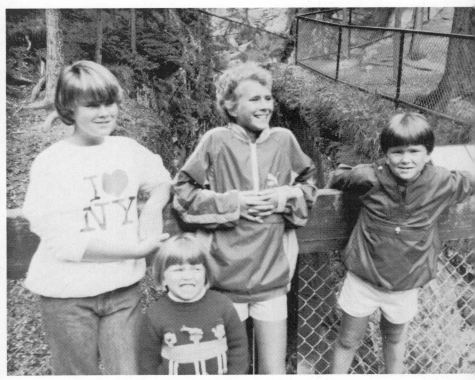

The Neuhaus kids in Canada, August 1984. From left:
Mary Kessler, Alexandra, Bo, and Charlie.

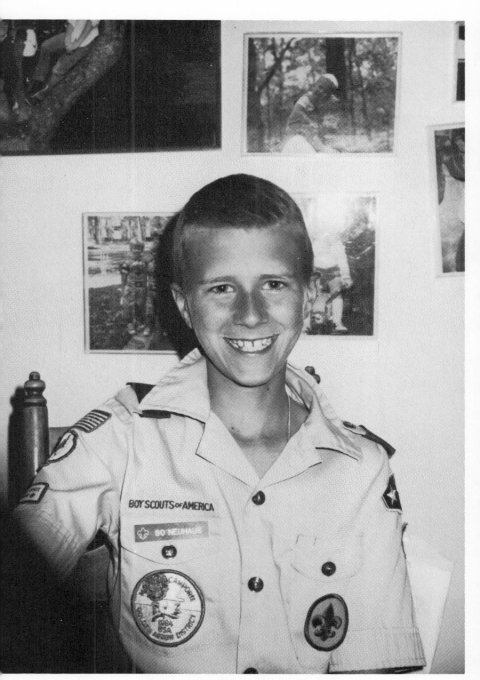

Scout Bo Neuhaus, Fall 1984

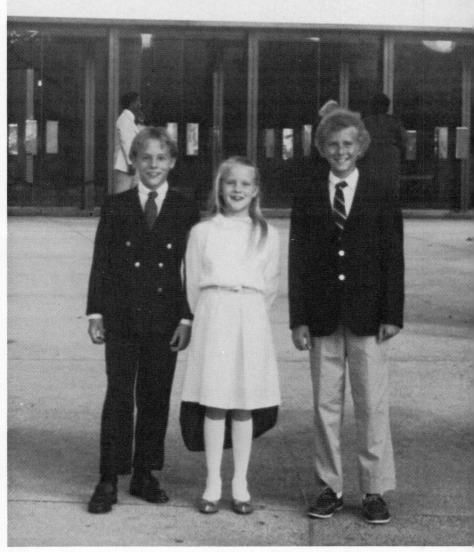

Bo with his friends George and Marcia Biggs at the
Don Francisco concert, September 1984.

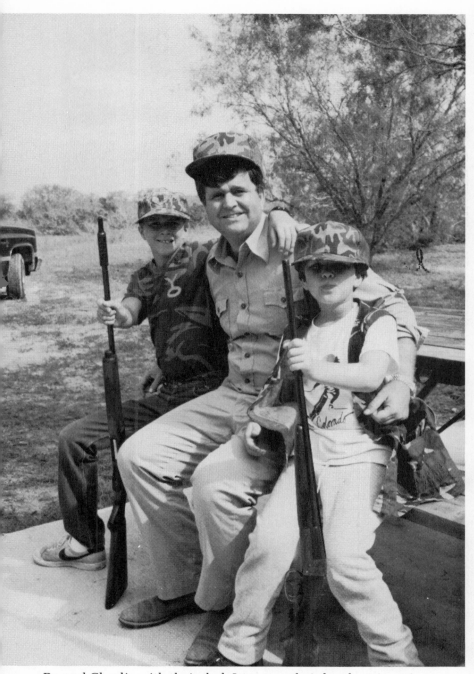

Bo and Charlie with their dad, Larry, on their last hunting trip together.

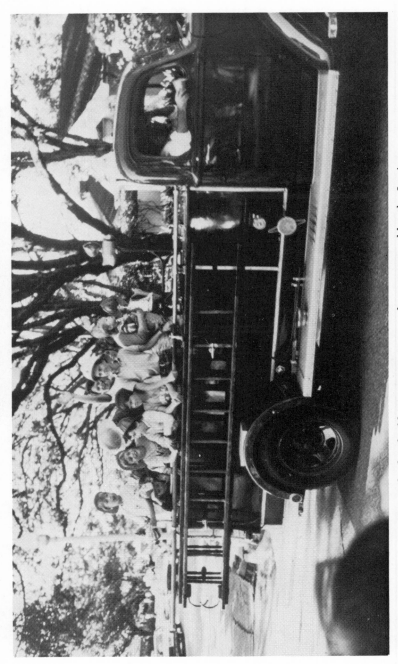

Bo at the lead of his very own parade, sponsored by the Junior League of Houston, November 1984.

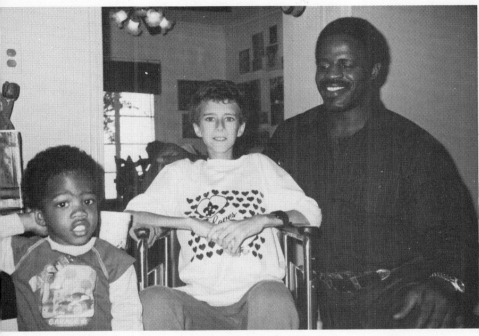

*Football star Earl Campbell and his son, Christian, paid Bo a
visit in early 1985.*

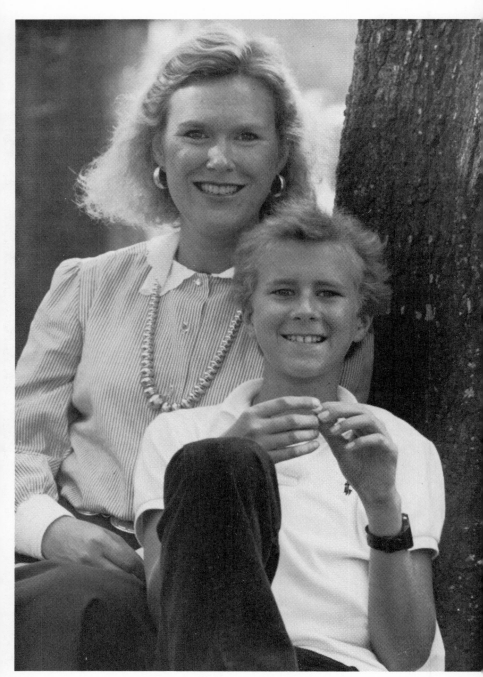

Lindy and Bo, October 1984